Class, Inequalities and Nursing Practice

Edited by

Margaret Miers

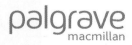
macmillan

First published 2003 by
PALGRAVE MACMILLAN
Houndmills, Basingstoke, Hampshire RG21 6XS and
175 Fifth Avenue, New York, N.Y. 10010
Companies and representatives throughout the world

PALGRAVE MACMILLAN is the global academic imprint of the Palgrave Macmillan division of St. Martin's Press, LLC and of Palgrave Macmillan Ltd. Macmillan® is a registered trademark in the United States, United Kingdom and other countries. Palgrave is a registered trademark in the European Union and other countries.

ISBN 0–333–96612–0 paperback

This book is printed on paper suitable for recycling and made from fully managed and sustained forest sources.

A catalogue record for this book is available from the British Library.

A catalog record for this book is available from the Library of Congress.

10   9   8   7   6   5   4   3   2   1
12 11 10 09 08 07 06 05 04 03
Printed in China

For David, John and Anne

Contents

Series editors' preface

It is widely accepted that because sociology can provide nurses with valuable and pertinent insights, it should be a constituent part of nursing's knowledge base. To take but a few substantive examples, sociology can help nurses understand the causes and distribution of ill health, the experience of health, illness and disability, the dynamics of health care encounters and the possibilities and limitations of professional care. Equally important, sociology's emphasis on critical reflection can encourage nurses to be more questioning and self-aware, thus helping them to provide flexible, non discriminatory, client-centred care in varied situations.

Unfortunately, while the aspiration of integrating sociology into nursing knowledge is easy enough to state in theory, in practice the relationship has not been as productive as some might have anticipated. Notwithstanding a number of works which have successfully applied sociological tools to nursing problems, there remains a gulf between the two disciplines which has led some to question the utility of the relationship.

On the one hand, sociologists, while taking an interest in nursing's occupational position, have not paid great attention to the actual work that nurses do. This is partially due to the limitations of sociological surveillance. Nurses work in confidential, private and intimate settings with their clients. Sociologists' access to such settings is necessarily restricted. Moreover, nurses find it difficult to talk about their work, except to other nurses. As a result, core issues pertaining to nursing have been less than thoroughly treated in the sociological literature. There is thus a disjunction between what nurses require from sociology and what sociologists can provide.

On the other hand, nurses are on equally uncertain ground when they attempt to use sociology themselves. Often nurses are reliant on carefully simplified introductory texts which, because of their broad remit, are often unable to provide in-depth understanding of sociological insights. Nor is it simply a matter of knowledge; there are tensions between the outlooks of nursing and sociology. Because nursing work involves individual interactions, it is not surprising that when nurses turn to sociology, they often turn to those elements which concentrate on micro-social interaction. While this is useful, in so far as it goes, it does not provide nurses with knowledge of the restraints and enablements imposed upon individual actions by social structures.

The aim of the *Sociology and Nursing Practice* series is to bridge these gaps between the disciplines. The authors of the series are nurses or teachers of nurses and therefore have an intimate understanding of nursing work and an appreciation of the importance of individualised nursing care. At the same time they are committed to a sociological outlook that asserts the salience of wider social forces to the work of nurses. The texts apply sociological theories and concepts to practical aspects of nursing. They explore nursing care as part of the social world, showing how different approaches to understanding the relationship between the individual and society have implications for nursing practice. By concentrating on specific concepts and drawing on research informed by social theory and methods, each book is able to provide the reader with a deeper understanding of the social construction of nurses' work. We hope the series will encourage nurses to analyse critically their practice and profession and to develop their own contribution to health and social care.

Margaret Miers, Sam Porter and Geoff Wilkinson

Acknowledgements

I owe thanks to family, friends and colleagues who have supported me during the preparation of this text. I am particularly grateful to Elaine, Paul, Robert and Valerie for contributing chapters, to Debra Salmon for editorial comments on Chapter Seven, and to all authors who have contributed to the development of the *Sociology and Nursing Practice Series*. Jon Reed has maintained the high standards of editorial guidance and tolerance practised by his predecessors. His support and that of my series editors Sam Porter and Geoff Wilkinson has been invaluable. My thanks to Geoff, who has found time, as ever, to read, review and reassure.

Chapter Eight contains material which has been published as Hoskins R and Carter D (2000) Welfare benefits screening and referral: A new direction for community nurses? *Health and Social Care in the Community* 8(6): 390–7 and appears by permission of Blackwell Publishers.

Margaret Miers

Notes on contributors

Elaine Denny is Head of Division, Health Policy and Sociology, School of Health and Policy Studies at the University of Central England in Birmingham. Her research interests focus around women as recipients and providers of health care, and she has published work on women's experience of IVF, and on the occupation of nursing. Her current research is on women's experience of living with endometriosis.

Paul Godin teaches research, community care and the historical sociology of mental health care at City University, the research area for his doctoral thesis. He is currently engaged in a qualitative research project examining the ideas and practice of risk assessment and risk reduction within forensic mental health services. Forthcoming publications include 'The frontline workforce of community mental health care' in Hannigan R, Coffey M and Burnard P (eds) *A Handbook of Community Mental Health Nursing*, Routledge, London.

Robert Hoskins is currently a Lecturer in the School of Nursing and Midwifery, University of Glasgow. Robert teaches health promotion, public health nursing, mental health and research methods. His main research interests are nurse-led welfare benefits uptake and public health nursing. He is currently working on research concerning the impact of a welfare benefit award on the perceived health status of the frail elderly.

Margaret Miers is Principal Lecturer, Faculty of Health and Social Care, University of the West of England, Bristol. She has overall responsibility for postgraduate research degree students within the Faculty and leads an Education Research and Development Unit. She also leads a research programme evaluating the Faculty's pre-qualifying interprofessional curriculum. She is series editor of Palgrave's *Sociology and Nursing Practice Series* and author of *Gender Issues and Nursing Practice* in the same series.

Valerie Watson is Senior Lecturer and Associate Head, Maternal and Child Health School, Faculty of Health and Social Care, University of the West of England, Bristol. Her teaching encompasses a range of child health issues, with a special interest in school nursing. Her research includes a scoping study of parenting activities in the South West.

Introduction

At a time of considerable change and development in the National Health Service, individual nurses and nursing as a profession face challenges and opportunities. Nurses are being offered opportunities to contribute to the public health workforce, to extend their roles in clinical practice, to learn and work in a range of health and social care teams and to develop their own judgment and decision making skills. They are being expected to reduce health inequalities and to improve equal access to health care. Nurses' educational preparation for the future remains a topic of debate. The Royal College of Nursing has pledged support for an all-graduate profession (Royal College of Nursing Presidential Taskforce on Nurse Education 2002) and is leading a consultation to agree a definition of nursing. In the *Defining Nursing* consultation report the authors note that contributors to the consultation emphasised 'know-how' knowledge, associated with personal experience, rather than 'know-that' knowledge, derived from theory and research. The report notes that in the United Kingdom nursing knowledge is seen as an 'amalgam', a melting pot, which provides the basis to support nurses' focus on individual patients and clients (Royal College of Nursing Defining Nursing Group 2002). This 'amalgam' approach to nursing knowledge is reflected in an 'integrated' approach to designing nursing curricula, which often leads to limited visibility for separate contributing disciplines such as sociology.

It will not be surprising that I have some difficulties with the 'amalgam' model, despite the fact that I see learning as an individual synthesis of knowing how and knowing that, creating new knowledge from often separate strands of enquiry. If in the melting pot we cannot see the difference and diversity of contributing bodies of knowledge, we may not understand and learn from the centrality and distinctiveness of the core concerns and core questions such disciplines ask themselves.

1

The studies of physiological, psychological and social processes respectively can be examined and understood on their own terms, through their own traditions. These separate processes warrant attention before nursing's 'glue' of individualised care becomes effective. The books in this series explore some of sociology's core concerns and questions about social processes in the belief that understanding these processes supports nursing in addressing its own core concerns.

Sociology's core concerns — power, gender, ethnicity, the division of labour, class and inequalities — are understood and explained differently by different theoretical traditions in sociology (Porter 1998). These traditions evolve, bringing new insights into the discipline. This series seeks to ensure that these new insights will find their way into nursing's melting pot. As nurses develop their role in public health it is likely that they will benefit from a deeper understanding of health interventions at community and policy level and of the theory and research which support these interventions. As Chapters One and Ten identify, all health professionals are being expected to contribute to the Government's agenda to reduce inequalities in health. They are also expected to provide equal access to equal services. As Hart and Lockey (2002: 486) have noted, however, there is a 'potential mismatch between policy visions and actual practice'. In their research into midwifery education and practice in relation to 'disadvantaged clients', Hart and Lockey found that policy visions are not followed through at operational level; different midwives worked with different concepts of disadvantage and managers 'did not have clear and specific strategies in relation to inequalities in health' (*ibid.*: 489). Midwifery and nursing's emphasis on individualised care does not necessarily prepare practitioners to appreciate the complexity and importance of processes of disadvantage, nor to recognise the limits as well as the possibilities of their own role. Greater clarity about strategic responsibility for identifying priorities for action in relation to inequalities in health may lead to role differentiation within nursing, with some nurses becoming public health specialists. All practitioners, however, have a responsibility to reflect on their own assumptions about inequalities in health. It is in the nature of social processes that all of us, at different times, feel disadvantaged and disempowered through the dynamics of social relationships as well as the rigidity of social structures. Learning from individual experience, however, is not an adequate knowledge base for assumptions about who is disadvantaged and why. Learning from relevant theories and research in combination with our own and others' individual experiences is a more effective basis for practice.

Writing this book has proved to be a vehicle for a deeper level of reflection, sometimes unexpected, about my own experience of social class. As a sociology undergraduate in the late 1960s I came to recognise the significance of my class background in my own life experience. I had thought that I had gained my place at university on the basis of my own individual achievements. An exploration of statistical data, summarised in the annual publication *Social Trends*, showed me that I was amongst a privileged minority. I began to see the deep significance of professional parents, material advantages, and of a selective school education. In the education hierarchy, a high position brought confidence and the higher education system itself deliberately encouraged and rewarded autonomy in use (or misuse) of time and thinking your own thoughts. Later, when gendered struggles to manage employment and caring responsibilities led me to train and work as a nurse, I was shocked to recognise the cultural significance of class based educational values (about autonomy and abstract thought) and the subtleties of societal devaluing of practical skills. As a student nurse I was embarrassed by the difficulties I had learning proficiency in practical skills. But I watched and learned from the social world of nursing, understanding the ritual, the hierarchy and the inequalities. In South Wales, I observed the long reach of industrial disease. Class inequalities in health, through all the mechanisms of material inequality, capitalist exploitation, cultural understandings and patterns of living, relations of dominance, subordination and submission, were part of the fabric of patients' experience and of my relationships with them. Class was also part of the fabric of my relationships within multiprofessional teams. Consultants could intimidate the student nurse but the middle class professional did not intimidate *me*. I expected civility and equality and sometimes found the confidence to negotiate it. But I also accepted my subordination, understanding very well the limits of my own relevant expertise. The effects of class on nursing's history is explored by Elaine Denny in Chapter Four; Paul Godin and Valerie Watson in Chapters Six and Seven respectively discuss how divisions within nursing have affected mental health nurses and children's nurses, contributing to the neglect of the interests of disadvantaged client groups. In Chapter Five, I explore the complicit role of education in perpetuating social hierarchies.

I have written this book to encourage nurses to understand and to explore the social processes which support and limit individual opportunities (including their own). Social processes limit and support opportunities for health. These processes at a societal level are linked to the division of labour as well as to the ownership of and access to resources. Chapter One explores these broad ideas, whereas later chapters discuss more specific explanations for the relationship between socio-economic status and health. Chapter Two introduces approaches to measuring the relationship between social class, health and illness and alerts the reader to a range of significant national and cohort studies that provide databases from which epidemiologists and health service researchers explore the complexity of associations between life events, circumstances and health. Chapter Three reviews the history of evidence and debate about health and inequalities. Robert Hoskins, in Chapter Eight, demonstrates how an understanding of debates and evidence around relative and absolute income led to an innovative approach to enabling community nurses to contribute to improving public health in Glasgow. Chapters Nine and Ten draw on broad and specific theories and relevant research to explore the role of nurses in occupational health and in public health and policy.

Throughout the book I have deliberately decided against including tables and figures which purport to provide the most up to date information concerning trends in mortality and morbidity. It is now possible to have easy access to a wide range of statistical and research based information that is more up to date than any textbook can hope to provide. The Department of Health website (www.doh.gov.uk) provides regular updates on its own monitoring of health inequality strategy and targets, and the Office for National Statistics

(ONS) provides web based updated information from the 2001 census and from Government surveys as well as downloadable publications such as *Social Trends,* an established reference source about the nature of British society with a commentary on relevant changes and trends. The virtual bookshelf on the Office for National Statistics website (www.statistics.gov.uk) lists morbidity and mortality statistics. By the time this text is published, mortality statistics by socioeconomic group using the 2001 census data may be available, thus providing further information for researchers to explore and debate. The research literature is also now readily available through databases which practitioners and students can access online through employers' and university resources as well as through the Royal College of Nursing. The *British Medical Journal* is also publicly accessible online (www.bmj.com). The internet challenges all of us to find and use information in different ways. It is tempting to think that the expansion of knowledge means we cannot synthesise information ourselves, but paradoxically, the internet means we can access *sources* of information more quickly. This means we can ensure that our synthesis rests on more reliable data sources, if we know where to find and how to use them. The challenge for nurses, and all professionals, is to become familiar with their own routes to information from research, from the Government, and from the professions and to use those routes regularly. We are able to critique and synthesise the information through asking questions that matter to us and to our clients. Why do babies born to manual workers have a lower life expectancy than babies born to parents working in professional jobs? Why and how does social class affect health? What health gains can be expected from changes in lifestyle, or from changes in levels of social support, or from changes in relative or absolute income levels? How can we measure such changes, and how can we measure health gains? These are all questions that matter to the Department of Health, the National Health Service, social scientists, health researchers, and, I hope, to nurses. This book is about these questions.

PART I

Explaining health inequalities

1 Understanding class and inequality

Margaret Miers

Introduction

In Britain, the beginning of a new century has been accompanied by the development of a programme of action to tackle inequalities in health. In 1998 the Government published the results of an inquiry into the nature and determinants of health inequalities in England. The recommendations of this *Independent Inquiry into Inequalities in Health*, chaired by Sir Donald Acheson, have subsequently been incorporated into many of the policy initiatives promoted to tackle inequalities in health, a priority area for the National Health Service (NHS) (Acheson 1998). In Autumn 2001 a national consultation took place on a plan to ensure that national targets for reducing health inequalities in England can be met. Similar initiatives in Wales and Scotland demonstrate governmental acceptance that not only do inequalities exist, but that 'many are avoidable and often unjust' (Department of Health (DoH) 2001a: 7). The injustice lies in the fact that 'such inequalities in health are a consequence of significant differences in opportunity, in access to services, and in material resources, as well as differences in personal lifestyle choices' (*ibid.*: 7).

It is the findings and arguments of the social scientists and health researchers who contributed to the *Independent Inquiry into Inequalities in Health* which are informing the Government's action plan. As the consultation document *Tackling Health Inequalities: Consultation on a Plan for Delivery* notes:

> To summarise these findings, people who experience one or more of: material disadvantage, lower educational attainment and/or insecure employment are likely to experience worse health than the rest of the population. In addition there is evidence to suggest that living in materially deprived neighbourhoods contributes to worse health for individuals.

These differences are apparent from the beginning of life. Children born and brought up in families with low levels of educational attainment, material disadvantage or in lower socio-economic groups are likely to experience worse health in later life. Although this country has seen increased prosperity and reductions in mortality, the gap in health between those at the top and bottom of the social scale has widened, particularly between the mid 1970s and the mid 1990s. This is significantly avoidable and fundamentally unfair. (DoH *op. cit.*: 7)

Behind the above analysis of health inequalities lies an implicit description of the nature of British society. It is presented as a differentiated society in which different individuals, families and groups share different experiences, particularly in relation to material and economic resources. Sociologists would describe such a society as stratified. Individuals are ranked by their access to resources. Individuals' position on 'the social scale' has implications for their health, and children's experiences early in life appear to influence their health at a later age. The British Government in the 21st century sees the negative health consequences of lack of access to adequate resources as both avoidable and unfair. The action plan to reduce health inequalities concentrates on two aims. The first is to reduce the gap in mortality between manual groups and the population as a whole, starting with children. The second is to reduce regional differences in life expectancy. A range of national targets are seen as central to achieving these aims. These are: reducing the number of children living in child poverty; reducing smoking rates, and reducing the under 18 conception rate. These targets indicate that the explanations offered for inequalities in health include explanations relating to income and material inequalities as well as explanations relating to behaviour and lifestyle. The results of the consultation further support the importance of tackling these factors, described as 'the wider determinants of health inequalities' (DoH 2002a: 8).

It is important to note that in suggesting that *health* inequalities are unfair and avoidable, the Government is not suggesting that *all* inequalities are unfair or capable of being eliminated. There is, however, an assumption that society has a responsibility for an individual's health. A review of different approaches to understanding and explaining inequalities in society provides the context for reviewing assumptions about societal and individual responsibility for health.

Social stratification

Sociology has traditionally used the concept of social stratification to explore inequality. Sociology textbooks, in chapters on social stratification, explain that all societies have divisions between people according to a hierarchical system, based usually on the amount of power and wealth individuals command (Giddens 1997, Haralambos and Holborn 2000). In some societies the divisions may be between age groups, gender, or ethnicity. In others, as in the Indian caste system, the divisions may be determined by religious beliefs. In industrialised societies the main basis of stratification has been socio-economic position, or, as sociologists have argued, social class. Up until the 1970s social class was commonly seen as the main form of social stratification in Britain, but since the 1970s there has been considerable debate about the importance of class in contemporary societies. Within sociology, Abbott and Wallace (1990) criticised the discipline for focussing too much on the male world of work and forgetting the importance of gender as a system of stratification. Throughout the 1980s and 1990s there has been a growing awareness of the importance of other differences between individuals and groups (Oliver 1990, Culley and Dyson 2001). Diversity and difference associated with ethnicity, sexual preference, ability and disability have led to both an interest in the complexity of social divisions and an emphasis on a growing individualisation of experience. Margaret Thatcher proclaimed 'There's no such thing as society' (hence no social structure, nor social stratification), and John Major's 'classlessness' was emphasised during his premiership; but sociologists, too, were pointing to the irrelevance of class as a concept in a world described by some as 'postmodern' (Featherstone 1991, Lash and Urry 1994). Social stratification involves the notion of a system, suggesting a structural determinism, which, it can be argued, fails to describe the pliable processes of social life. Touraine (1995) has argued that sociology needs concepts to describe fluidity rather than structure and suggests that social movements, not social class, should be a central category of sociological analysis.

All health professionals involved in implementing *The NHS Plan* (DoH 2000) face the challenge of understanding the nature and genesis of health inequalities, which the present Labour Government acknowledges as avoidable and unfair. Exploring notions of social stratification, social class and social diversity and social movement, is part of that challenge.

Is inequality inevitable?

The view that some form of stratification is inevitable, or just, has a long history. In ancient Greece, slavery was perceived as natural for slaves and assumptions about women's inferiority to men have only been challenged through legislation in the 20th century. Feudalism accepted and supported material inequalities between serfs and lords. The Hindu caste system is an obvious example of inequality being seen as divinely ordained. However the idea that human beings are born equal developed during the 17th century, alongside attempts to articulate the relationship between an individual and the state as a representation of a collectivity. Political theorists such as Hobbes (1588–1679), Locke (1632–1704) and Rousseau (1712–78) argued that democratic political systems would allow the authority of the state to protect individual rights. These changes were accompanied by industrialisation and the growth of capitalism, a process which many sociologists describe as leading to 'modernity', characterised by the growth of organisations, industry and capitalism (Crompton 1998). Social class became the dominant form of social stratification in this period of 'modernity'. There are many definitions of social class but all involve an understanding of ranked collectivities of people sharing a measure of prestige or resources. These unequal shares can be seen as fair or unfair, avoidable or unavoidable, depending on explanations for the distribution and accrual of these resources.

Functionalist theories of stratification

Functionalists argued that resources are distributed in a manner which maintains social stability. Functionalism, as an approach to understanding how society works, draws on a biological analogy and describes society as a social system made up of interrelated parts. Different 'parts' of society contribute to the maintenance of the order and stability of society as a whole. Social stratification, therefore, is functional for the integrated social system. Talcott Parsons (1951) believed that order and stability are based on consensus about what is valued in society and that value consensus is the basis of cooperation and integration within society. Evaluation of activities, skills and individuals is based on the consensus of the group and those who successfully perform highly valued activities will be held in high regard. The resulting status and prestige are usually accompanied by material rewards. Stratification and inequality are a means of reinforcing common values and thus help maintain social stability. Davis and Moore (1945) gave the most detailed account of how social stratification supports the effective functioning of social systems. They argued that all societies need a mechanism for ensuring that key roles are effectively allocated and performed. The most important roles in society must be filled by those best able to perform them. The most able individuals must receive appropriate training and the most important roles must be performed conscientiously. The promise of high rewards ensures that the most able individuals are attracted to the most important social roles. Such assumptions may underlie the allocation of professional roles. Davis and Moore argue that social stratification is a device by which societies ensure that the most able and qualified persons gain the most important positions. (For a summary and critique of this position in relation to the allocation of professional roles, see Wilkinson and Miers 1999.)

Davis and Moore's functionalist account of the inevitability of social stratification has been widely criticised, most comprehensively by Tumin. Tumin (1964) noted that many occupations which are vital to society (hospital domestic, refuse collector, to name but two) are not valued and occupy a low position in a stratification system. He questioned the view that there is only a limited pool of individuals with the ability to perform some highly valued roles and the view that training for key positions involved sacrifice, given that the long term rewards of higher education were well known. Tumin argued that Davis and Moore had ignored the influence of power in the allocation of prestige and resources, suggesting that those groups occupying highly rewarded positions can restrict access to their positions through controlling entry, thus creating demand for their own scarce skills and thereby increasing their own rewards. High status professions such as the medical profession are offered as exemplars of the self interested use of power. Stratification could therefore serve as inhibiting individual development and opportunity and serve to divide, not integrate, social groups.

Many commentators on functionalist theories of stratification have noted that:

> such theories incorporate a moral justification of economic inequality which has been commonplace since the advent of economic liberalism — that is, in a competitive market society, it is the most talented and ambitious — in short the best that get to the top, and therefore take the greater part of societies' rewards. (Crompton 1998: 7)

The moral justification includes the view that an individual's social position is an individual's responsibility. Similarly, individuals are responsible for their own health. This moral justification, however, is often based on assumptions about equality of opportunity, which as Crompton points out 'is a powerful justification for inequality' (*op. cit.*: 7). Governments can take measures to increase equality of opportunity through limiting the power of those with control over resources by various regulatory devices such as legislation against monopolies and legislation to protect employees. A further force that mitigates the divisiveness of stratification and promotes equality of opportunity is the development of social citizenship, that is, universal provision of education and welfare benefits. The current Government's attention to inequalities in health can be viewed as an attempt to reaffirm a commitment to equality of access to health and health care for all citizens. Such a commitment is enshrined in the values of the NHS and the Labour Government's concern is to identify the barriers to equal access to health care. In so far as the barriers are economic barriers, these are identified and action to address them is part of the action plan for tackling health inequalities. National policies outside of the NHS identified as being directed towards reducing health inequalities include:

● continuing to improve the position of the poorest working families by increasing the National Minimum Wage

- reducing the risk of ill health and excess winter deaths among older and disabled people by implementing *The UK Fuel Poverty Strategy*
- addressing the housing needs of deprived areas by bringing all social housing up to set standards of decency by 2010 (DoH 2001a: 26).

This is not, however, a challenge to Britain's economic reward system.

Marx on social class

Karl Marx (1818–83) saw inequality as inevitable within capitalism. He saw capitalism as a social system characterised by private ownership of wealth. Sociologists in the 1960s and 1970s explored the writings of Marx as a radical alternative to functionalism. He observed that human beings must produce food and material objects in order to survive and to do so individuals develop social relationships with each other. As the 'forces of production', that is the raw materials, knowledge and tools used in production, develop, so will social relationships, the relations of production, change and develop. Groups come to occupy different positions in relation to the forces and relations of production, leading to an inevitable conflict of interests between social groups. This conflict of interests derives from a contradiction between the forces and the relations of production and class conflict becomes the driver of historical change. The forces and relations of production together form the economic base or infrastructure of society and the infrastructure shapes the ideas and values of society, including the structures supporting these ideas and values — the legal and political system, education, health and welfare services. Hence far from social structure and stratification being based on consensus, they are based on conflictual economic relationships between oppositional social groups. It is the ideas of those with the most economic power, which become the accepted, consensual ideas.

The oppositional social groups are classes. Marx and Engels, in *The Communist Manifesto*, proclaimed:

> The history of all hitherto existing society is the history of class struggles. Freeman and slave, patrician and plebeian, lord and serf, guild

master and journeyman, in a word, oppressor and oppressed, stood in constant opposition to one another, carried on an uninterrupted, now hidden, now open fight, a fight that each time ended either in a revolutionary reconstitution of society at large, or in the common ruin of the contending classes. (Marx and Engels 1967: 79)

In capitalist societies the capitalists (the bourgeoisie) own the means of production and the workers (the proletariat) own only their own labour which they hire to the employers (the bourgeoisie) in return for wages. The capitalist employer sells the products for more than the costs of the labour and the materials and the surplus value constitutes the capitalist's profit. As Crompton (1998) explains, although human labour is unique, in that it has the capacity to create new value by transforming commodities, in a capitalist society labour has become a commodity like any other. It is purchased as a raw material for a price that does not take account of its transformative capacity to create new value. Thus it is in the interests of the employer to control the wages and in the interests of the worker to increase levels of pay. There is a contradiction between the forces of production (the 'material' used in production plus the collective labour power of the workers) and the relations of production (private and individual ownership and individual wage payments). The interests of workers as a collectivity are in conflict with the system of private and individual ownership. The conflict between the two opposed classes, Marx predicted, would lead, through revolutionary means, to the final epoch of history, a communist or socialist society in which the forces of production (collective labour) would be congruent with the relations of production, through collective ownership. Class conflict, oppression and exploitation would be eliminated. Contradiction would be resolved. It was the injustice in class relations which would lead to the ending of inequality.

Porter (1998) has illustrated the relevance of Marxism to nursing by reference to Bridges and Lynam's (1993) Marxist analysis of informal carers. Bridges and Lynam identify ways in which the logic of capitalism affects the lives of informal carers. In a Marxist analysis, public expenditure (for example expenditure on the NHS) is a significant drain on profit and it is 'therefore in the interests of the capitalist economic sector to ensure that public expenditure is kept to a minimum' (Porter *op. cit.*: 55). Bridges and Lynam interpret the move towards community care, relying on unpaid informal labour, as a move to reduce public expenditure, reflecting capital's economic need to maximise profits. This economic need leads the producers of the goods (and services) that lead to profit to keep down costs and maintain their own structural position in the capitalist economic system. In health care it is the professionals who are the producers of the services and it is in their own interests to retain their economic position by neglecting the interests of service users and informal carers. Porter notes:

> given that carers tend to be disadvantaged and unsupported within the economic and social circumstances currently pertaining, there is likely to be a gulf between the needs of the carer and the ideology of the ruling class. Here we come to nurses' dilemma of whether to act as an advocate, promoting the needs and desires of their clients, or to act in the interests of the bureaucracy for which they work. (Porter *op. cit.*: 56)

A Marxist analysis challenges nurses to acknowledge their own position in the stratification system and the implications of their own mode of professional practice. Nurses may also wish to consider whether their own labour has transformative power, capable of creating new value through improving health. Such a claim, if it can be made good, can be an argument for higher rewards. Godin, in Chapter Six in this volume, analyses the position of mental health nursing within the capitalist context of mental health policy and practice.

Max Weber and social stratification

Marx was not the only social theorist, of course, to write about class. Max Weber (1864–1920) also saw class as an economic grouping and defined class as a group of individuals who share a similar position in the market economy and as a result gain similar economic rewards. Individuals who share a market position share a class position. The highest economic rewards will go to those who have capital, property and skills which can be used, in Marx's terms, as part of the forces of production. Market position depends on scarcity; highly valued and scarce professional skills (in medicine, the law) would attract high rewards. It is relevant to note that Weber's analysis has been used to explain the professional closure strategies used to protect professionals' market position (Johnson 1972, Witz 1992). Weber, however, disagreed with Marx's view that social status and political power derive from economic power. Weber identified three separate dimensions of stratification: class, status and party. He saw all three as phenomena of the distribution of power within a community:

> Whereas the genuine place of classes is within the economic order, the place of status groups is within the social order, that is, within the sphere of the distribution of honour. From within these spheres, classes and status groups influence one another and the legal order and are in turn influenced by it. 'Parties' reside in the sphere of power. Their action is oriented toward the acquisition of social power, that is toward influencing social action no matter what its content may be. (Weber 1995 [1978]: 39)

To Weber, therefore, inequality has many dimensions. It is neither just nor unjust but an inevitable feature of society.

Functionalists, Marx and Weber are often described as constituting the classical tradition in sociology. These theorists have, as Roberts (2001) suggests, established the common denominators of any description of society that adopts a class analysis. All 'are agreed that classes have an economic foundation: they are composed of people with common experiences of making their livings. So people are invariably "classed" on the basis of their occupations' (Roberts *op. cit.*: 6). All would also agree that class matters. In health, it certainly appears that it does. Although life expectancy rose for all social groups between 1970 and 1996, life expectancy for men in social class 1 (professional and managerial) increased by 5.7 years but the gain amongst men in social class 5 (unskilled manual) was only 1.7 years (Hattersley 1999).

This does not mean that other social divisions such as ethnicity and gender do not matter. Economic differences, however, cross cut other inequalities, sometimes ameliorating and sometimes deepening disadvantage. This book is primarily about class and economic inequalities. Other books in the Sociology and Nursing Practice Series have explored other dimensions of stratification (Godfrey 1999, Miers 2000, Culley and Dyson 2001).

Class consciousness

Class theorists also share an assumption that class is not just an economic grouping. Class means something to individuals. Individual men and women identify themselves as belonging to a class and as sharing interests with those in the same economic grouping. Functionalists would see individuals in all social classes as sharing views about the meaning and fairness of the reward system which differentiates life experiences. Weber saw classes not as 'communities' but as possible bases for social action through shared 'economic interests in the possession of goods and opportunities for income' (Weber *op. cit.*: 32). For Weber, class situation is market situation and individuals may join together to preserve their market situation but this is not inevitable. Perceived membership of status groups, for example, may inhibit collective action. This is an issue which has been extensively discussed in the literature on race and class (Castles and Kozack 1973). Status divisions between majority and minority ethnic groups within Britain may have inhibited recognition of shared economic interests amongst unskilled workers.

Marx saw classes as social forces providing the means and momentum for historical change. He distinguished between the objective conditions of social classes, created by a group's relationship to the means of production, and the subjective sense of belonging to a class and sharing class identity and interests. He distinguished between 'class-in-itself' — a group whose members share an economic position — and 'class-for-itself' — a group whose members share class consciousness and a sense of solidarity. A group becomes united, 'and constitutes itself as a class-for-itself. The interests it defends become class interests. But the struggle of class against class is a political struggle' (Marx and Engels 1995: 29). Marx anticipated that the political struggle between the proletariat and the bourgeoisie would result in revolutionary change and the development of a communist society that, through collective ownership of the means of production, would abolish the conditions which created social classes. All theorists see connections between class and politics. Marx saw classes as *deriving* from relations of power and hence inevitably part of the political process.

Functionalists saw the linking of higher classes with higher levels of prestige and influence as inevitable. Weber saw class and parties as separate but recognised that market position could be a position to be protected and that parties, as political groups, could be representing class interests or status interests. The protection of the market situation through the creation of organisations to serve as professional groups with political influence, such as the British Medical Association and the Royal College of Nursing, has been a feature of professional activity in Britain.

Classes as contemporary and historical phenomena

It should be made clear that it is not only sociologists who have discussed class at considerable length. It is significant that Marx wrote some of his major works while living in Britain, and Engels' observations of working class life in northern England shaped his ideas and writings (Engels 1969 [1844]). British class divisions and class consciousness have been seen by other countries as a defining characteristic of the British nation, although it is often unclear whether what is being observed are, in Weber's or Marx's terms, class divisions, or an awareness of status distinctions. Devine (1997) has looked at the reality of class inequalities in Britain and the United States, arguing that there have been stereotypical assumptions about Britain being a class-bound society in contrast to the United States' classlessness. She concluded that both stereotypes are misleading although class identification has had a greater influence on political attitudes and behaviour in Britain than in America. Economic restructuring has reduced the size of the working class in Britain and in both countries there has been a growth in poverty. Her conclusion that 'social class has proved remarkably resilient over the twentieth century' (*ibid*.: 264) would be supported by Roberts (2001).

Historians, as well as sociologists, have viewed Britain as a class society and have analysed its development in class terms. Thompson (1968) has adopted a Marxist approach, arguing that class is a historical category and inseparable from notions of class struggle. He traces the development of the working class back through the 18th century. McKibbin (1990) explores the puzzle that despite the fact that 'in 1901 about 85 percent of the total working population were employed by others, and about 75 percent as manual workers', suggesting that 'in the broadest sense Britain was unquestionably a working-class nation' (*ibid*.: 2), there was no strong Marxist party in Britain. McKibbin explains this by the nature of the political system and the role of the state. The development of the National Health Service, for example, as part of the welfare state, can be seen as fostering shared values and shared culture despite economic inequalities. In recent decades economic change has been seen as resulting in the decline of the working class and a growth of the middle class, with a consequent diminution of differences between political parties seeking to represent public interests. Despite this, some writers identify continuing links between economic and political power (Scott 1997).

Class in decline?

The possible irrelevance of class in explaining inequalities, social diversity and social processes warrants careful consideration. Roberts (*op. cit.*) notes that class can be said to be in decline if one or more of three things happen. 'First, there would be a decline in class if occupations ceased to be arranged in "clumps" ' (*ibid*.: 12), that is, there is no grouping of occupations according to market position or in terms of relations of production. Second, class would be irrelevant if occupations had no significance in individuals' minds, that is, there is no consciousness of class situation. Third, class would cease to exist if 'the clustering of occupations, and the associated forms of consciousness (and unconsciousness), were insulated from politics' (*ibid*.: 12). He concludes his book on *Class in Modern Britain* by claiming that 'class analysis has been, and still is, the key to understanding the links between the economy, politics and society, how these have changed in the past, and the alternative ways in which they might change in the future' (*ibid*.: 251).

A fourth reason for the decline of class, however, could be if the clustering of occupations ceased to be linked to individual life chances. As Chapter Three of this volume demonstrates, however, class appears to remain closely linked to individual chances of lifetime experience of good or poor health.

Arguments about the decline in the significance of class include the embourgeoisement thesis, that is the argument that as manual workers earn more money they adopt the lifestyle of the bourgeoisie (Goldthorpe *et al.* 1969, Saunders 1990a,b). Margaret Thatcher's Conservative governments of 1979–90 can be seen as having encouraged this through encouraging the purchase of former local authority owned homes and the widespread purchasing of shares through privatisation of state owned industries and the conversion of building societies into banks. A further argument suggesting a reduced significance of class and economic inequality is the development of a form of citizenship (Marshall 1963) which includes rights to a minimum income, to educational opportunities, to health care and to adequate housing. The development of this social citizenship has been pursued by a range of disadvantaged groups including women, minority ethnic groups, lesbians and gay men, disabled people and users of mental health services. Chapter Six discusses citizenship in relation to mental health nursing. The defence and extension of citizenship can be seen as crossing the boundaries of class or other social divisions, thus limiting the importance of particular economic groups. Additionally, social mobility is seen as limiting the significance of class by breaking down class barriers, although research into health inequalities (see Chapter Three) suggests that class of origin can have a lifetime significance for health (Blane 1999, Benzeval *et al.* 2000).

Postmodernism and class

A more fundamental critique of the relevance of class comes from arguments which suggest that class was a feature of modern industrial societies and that in postindustrial, postmodern societies, class ceases to be significant. The decline in labour intensive mining and manufacturing suggests that labour power is no longer as important as technological power, and consumption, not production, becomes significant in influencing an individual's identity and lifestyle. There is an increasing diversity of opportunity available through varied economic and cultural positions. Waters (1997), for example, argues that from 1975 to the present, intelligence and marketable attributes have become more important than material property; status groups differentiated by lifestyle more important than class, and cultural identity more important than material inequality. This 'status conventionalism' (Pakulski and Waters 1996) is underway through an increasing individualism resulting from economic globalisation, a process which reduces national control over the economy and thus leads to a postmodern society characterised by what Beck (1992: 127) has termed 'a categorical shift' in the relationship between individual and society. Beck argues that individual ability to manage one's life in a 'risk' society has become more important than class position. Lash and Urry (1994) have argued that in the late stage of what they term 'disorganised capital', 'flows' of people, ideas, information, images, and capital are more important than structures, and culture rather than economic position brings meaning to self aware, reflexive individuals who shape and transform production and structure. For these writers, postmodern society is characterised by 'instability, fragmentation, individualization and social fluidity' (Crompton 1998: 131) and consumption is society's driving force. Nevertheless within the 'economies of signs and space' (Lash and Urry *op. cit.*) are conflicts and inequalities. These ideas, particularly the emphasis on culture, have suggested new ways of exploring and understanding social forces which lead to significant inequalities in health.

Bourdieu and types of capital

The French sociologist, Pierre Bourdieu's work has become influential in Britain, particularly through his inextricable linking of economic and social/cultural worlds in his formulation of the dynamic structuring of practice (Bourdieu 1977). Different conditions of existence are not separate from the perceptions and organising practices of those conditions. To discuss this, Bourdieu uses two terms, 'field' and 'habitus'. 'Field' is a structural system of social relations at a macro and micro level (such as the division of labour in health care). 'Habitus' is both the structured relations and the structuring process expressed through knowledge and action. Habitus is 'a structured and structuring structure':

> The habitus is not only a structuring structure, which organises prac-
> tices and perceptions of practices, but also a structured structure: the
> principle of division into logical classes which organises the percep-
> tion of the social world is itself the product of internalisation of the
> division into social classes. Each class condition is defined, simultane-
> ously, by its intrinsic properties and by the relational properties which
> it derives from its position in the system of class conditions,
> which is also a system of differences, differential positions. (Bourdieu
> 1986: 170–1)

Unlike Marx, Bourdieu sees class as indivisible from consciousness of class. Bourdieu also, significantly, identifies four different 'forms of capital' — economic, cultural, social and symbolic — which, as Crompton identifies, 'together empower (or otherwise) agents in the struggle for position within "social space"' (Crompton *op. cit.*: 148). Bourdieu sees classes as developing as a consequence of these empowerments. He uses the term 'class' as a general term for many social groups, sharing types of capital. Classes occupy a similar habitus. He is interested in the emergence of new groups and as such his views have been used to examine the emergence of new middle class groups developing through the growth of administrative, professional and managerial occupations. Within the literature on health inequalities, however, it is the role of social capital, loosely defined as involving 'connections, networks and group membership' (Anthias 2001: 841), which has attracted attention.

Putnam *et al.*'s (1993) study of engagement in community life in different regions of Italy has informed Wilkinson's (1996a,b) important analysis of inequality and health. Wilkinson has argued that health tends to be less good among populations where there are greater income differences, suggesting a link between relative deprivation and poorer health (see Chapters Three, Eight and Nine in this volume). The *perception* of inequality and injustice may lead to further inequality through physical effects on health. Putnam found that income inequality/equality was related to his index of 'civic community'. Equality is supportive of civic community, but civic community declines if income inequality increases. Wilkinson (1999) has argued that analysis by Kawachi *et al.* (1997), showing that trust in others declines where income inequalities are bigger, suggests a 'pathway from income distribution through quality of social relations to health' (*op. cit.*: 261). Income inequality constrains connections and networks within and across groups. A hierarchical and unequal system of income and status distribution, as Wilkinson *et al.* (1998) have argued, cuts people off from the respect accorded to high status and leads to sensitivity about status issues, and readiness to defend one's own position rather than support others. These ideas are reviewed extensively by Wilkinson (1996a, 1999) who argues that the stresses of hierarchy, hierarchical relations and structures of power and subordination are passed downwards with the result that 'friendships and social networks atrophy as people feel increasingly vulnerable to the way they are seen by others' (Wilkinson 1999: 267). This emphasis on the influence of the psychosocial environment on health, however, has prompted considerable debate (Lynch *et al.* 2000), discussed in Part Three of this volume.

Social exclusion

Interest in social cohesion and health is matched by concern about social exclusion and the possible development of an underclass. Such concern derives from the recognition that during the 1980s the political climate in Britain and the United States, led by Margaret Thatcher in Britain, drew on market approaches to economic management, disdaining Keynesian manipulation of the economy through government tax and investment schemes. The effect of the emphasis on the market as a way to regulate individual opportunities and income was a growing polarisation in income distribution. In 1999, Byrne claimed that:

> in the UK the real incomes of the lowest decile after housing costs were taken into account are now substantially below their value of 1979, having declined by some 25 per cent ... the top decile of incomes in contrast saw an increase of more than 60 per cent. (Byrne 1999: 81, see also Westergaard 1995: 132–3, Goodman *et al.* 1997: 112)

Those in the lowest decile are disproportionately in areas of the country hitherto dependent on mining and manufacturing (South Wales, the North East of England), in which young people, particularly young men, struggle to find permanent employment. Governments in the 1980s and 1990s supported the growth of the flexible labour market and reduced the tax burden on the affluent, with the intention of increasing the supply of jobs. The benefits system has not contributed to a redistribution of income.

Within cities, there has been concern that spatial divides have contributed to social exclusion through building projects of urban regeneration which have disrupted working class communities already disempowered by the decline of manufacturing work. Byrne (*op. cit.*) argues that to understand the nature and significance of social exclusion it is important to understand the change in the nature of social life in postindustrial capitalism in the 1980s and 1990s. Whereas during a period of growth from the mid 19th century until the 1970s, standards of living rose, in the 1980s and 1990s individuals felt considerably less secure. Post the Second World War, full employment, welfare benefits and strong trade unions ensured rising standards for all workers. More recently the emphasis has been on personal skills and flexibility to maintain one's position in the labour market. Social exclusion is seen as relating to those marked with personal deficits. In a market economy, there is no demand for their labour. Just as slaves could be seen as an underclass, in Marxist terms, since they did not own their own labour and thus had no position in the relations of production, so could some individuals be seen as falling into an underclass since they lack all forms of capital. The term 'underclass', however, has also been used by writers who have emphasised cultural factors which maintain the separation of social groups. Murray (1990, 1994) has argued that the poor develop a fatalism about their position in the world which reduces the capacity for self help. The importance of the term 'social exclusion' lies in its emphasis not on the behaviour of individuals or the culture of groups, but on the rights and entitlements that all citizens should have. The exclusion of some individuals from citizenship rights threatens all of us. As Crompton notes, 'the defence of citizenship, therefore, cuts across the boundaries of social class' (1998: 201). Department of Health policies to improve services for people with learning disabilities and for those with mental illness can be seen as attempts to develop services on a more inclusive basis (DoH 1999b, 2001b). In Chapter Six, Paul Godin considers the significance of citizenship and social exclusion in the care of people with mental illness.

Realism and the persistence of class

Scambler and Higgs (1999) maintain that 'real class relations' persist in Britain in the sense that class is real because of the relationships between persons. This is a position similar to Marx but deriving from Bhaskar's (1989) critical realism, a philosophical approach which recognises, as Porter (1998) explains, 'that there are objects of knowledge that exist independently of our thoughts' (*ibid.*: 171). Class relationships continue to hinge on relationships of ownership and control of the means of production. The realist approach to understanding social structure and social action accepts that social structures (such as relations of production) impose constraints and enablements on individuals' freedom to act in their own interests. Realism, however, does not see economic relations as of prime importance as Marx argued. Social structures such as patriarchy also affect relationships between persons. In open social systems different structures affect action, thus bringing choice not constraint; nevertheless social reality is not grounded in individual consciousness. Class may not be central to individual experience but its significance remains real.

The importance of class relationships as underlying factors in the causal pathways to inequalities in health remains a topic of considerable debate. The relationships between groups in a social structure have consequences for individuals' material circumstances (housing, income, access to services and amenities) and for their sense of security, social position and self worth. Later chapters discuss the significance of material pathways and psychosocial pathways in determining health through considering the evidence and arguments of health inequality researchers. Discussions of underlying social processes, through arguments about postmodernism or realism, lie in the domain of sociology, with its responsibility to observe general processes of social cohesion, social differentiation and social stratification.

Conclusion

This chapter has introduced a range of approaches to understanding social class and inequality. The different approaches provide different answers to questions which are central to an understanding of social stratification and of nurses' position in a social hierarchy. Relevant questions include: how do the skills individuals have and the work individuals do relate to their social status and their position in a social class hierarchy? How do economic resources relate to work and skill? Do economic resources relate to the processes of wealth creation in types of social structures? To understand the significance of social class and nursing practice, nurses need to consider both their own class position and the position of their clients. Hugman (1991) helps explain the position of nursing and other caring professions amongst the middle class. Although caring professionals are selling their emotional and manual labour for income in a way that connects them to the working class, their professional education, 'career patterns and work autonomy (so far as that has been achieved) all serve to separate these occupations from the working class' (*ibid.*: 127). It is the claims to knowledge that establish class position and legitimise professional power. If knowledge is clearly demarcated, professional power is greater and is not dependent on organisational position. Hence doctors and lawyers have particularly clear professional status, partly through their ability to practise independently. Hugman argues that 'where the demarcation of an area of knowledge is weak then the organisational position is made more explicit' (*ibid.*: 128). It has been the organisational basis of employment that has preserved the power of nurses and caring professionals over clients. Power derived from knowledge and from organisational position has been buttressed by what Hugman terms 'ideological power', a process which shapes the images and meanings concerning client/professional relationships. Caring professionals maintain their own status and economic interests by placing the client in a disadvantaged position. If health inequalities result in a majority of service users coming from lower social classes, it is easy for caring professionals to maintain a social distance from their clients, a social distance which can sustain the professional's self image and stigmatise the user (as incompetent, irresponsible or immoral).

In recent years, however, there have been considerable challenges to professional power, from the users of services, from policy and from challenges to professional boundaries. Within this context, health inequalities and professionals' responsibilities to contribute to their reduction are receiving considerable attention. The challenge for nurses is to understand their own position within the stratification system and the implications of this for self and others. This book suggests that our material resources, our employment and our class relationships can affect the health of all of us, as professionals and as service users. Part One looks particularly at the evidence for the social determinants of health; Part Two looks at nursing's position in the class system and the factors that influence this; and Part Three encourages nurses to consider their own role and responsibilities in recognising the significance of clients' positions in relation to resources for health, and finding ways of enhancing not reducing those resources.

2 Measuring class and researching health inequalities

Margaret Miers

Introduction

Our understanding of the relationship between class, inequality and health depends on the ways in which we measure differences between people. It also depends on the information we gather when looking at the effects of economic inequalities and lifestyle differences on health and illness.

The most common approach to identifying social class position has been to take a person's occupation as a measure of their social class. Such an approach takes an 'objective' approach to measuring social class, ignoring the subjective views of the individuals assigned to particular groups. There are disadvantages in this approach. In my experience, for example, student nurses are often surprised to find they are identified as being in a relatively high position on a social class ranking. They do not feel they are in an advantageous position relative to other occupations, either in terms of social status or in terms of financial rewards. 'Objective' approaches to measuring social class have the main advantage of being easy to use and, in Britain, a considerable amount of information using social class rankings has been routinely collected by the Government and by researchers in order to monitor and understand demographic and social structure and change. Information about social class and health is routinely collected. The Office for National Statistics produces regular reports relevant to health, morbidity and mortality. Reports are available online on the Government statistics 'virtual bookshelf' (www.statistics.gov.uk). Information about social class, health and disease will become available on this website as data from the 2001 census are analysed. A significant text reporting on the results of studies funded under the

Health Variations research programme funded by the Economic and Social Research Council (Graham 2000a) includes information on standardised mortality ratios (SMRs) by social class; information about social class and heart disease and social class and lung function as well as information about income and health and varied approaches to measuring deprivation.

The Registrar General's definition of social class

The model of social class most familiar to health researchers is the Registrar General's classification of social class which was first used in the analysis of the 1911 census and has only recently been replaced by a revised scheme, the National Statistics Socio-Economic Classification (NS-SEC). As Graham (2000b) notes, this was developed to 'capture the pecking order of power, property and prestige; a pecking order in which women and children earned their place indirectly, through the occupation of the 'man of the house' (*ibid.*: 4). Recognition of these limitations has led to alternative approaches (discussed later in the chapter) which are more successful in describing women's class position.

The Registrar General's classification of social class divided the population into six social classes based on the occupation of the head of the household. Occupations were grouped together into the scheme with the aim of ensuring that:

> as far as is possible, each category is homogeneous in relation to the general standing within the community of the occupations concerned. This criterion is naturally correlated with ... other factors such as education and economic environment, but it has no direct relationship to the average level of remuneration of particular occupations. (Central Statistical Office 1966: xiii)

The descriptions of the six classes varied slightly over the decades. The descriptions used in analysis of the 1991 census are listed below:

- Class I   Professional
- Class II   Managerial and technical
- Class IIINM   Skilled non-manual

- Class IIIM   Skilled manual
- Class IV   Partly skilled
- Class V   Unskilled

The strengths of the Registrar General's classification rest on the fact that it was used for most of the 20th century, providing continuity in the way data have been collected about Britain's changing class structure. Much of our information about persistence and change in health inequalities relies on this continuity. In fact the impetus to develop and use the scheme came from interest in levels of infant mortality. It was developed at a time of debate about hierarchies of natural ability and social hierarchies (Szreter 1984). One of the criticisms of the Registrar General's classification was that it relied too unquestioningly on hierarchies of social prestige (general standing in the community) and hence was not an adequate reflection of the relative earning power of occupations. As a scale it could be seen as relying too much on 'subjective' judgments about status rather than 'objective' economic position. Furthermore, difficulties in classifying particular occupations led to regular revisions. In 1961, for example, postmen were reclassified, moving from class III to class IV; the category of 'manager' has posed difficulties and changing and developing occupations such as airline pilots and computer programmers have been allocated or reallocated to a category without any research to support the categorisation (Crompton 1998, Roberts 2001). The boundary between manual and non-manual work was particularly difficult to identify as many occupations include both manual and non-manual workers. From 1981, the Registrar General's department identified skill, rather than social standing, as a main basis for the classification of social class but occupations were not reclassified according to skill rather than status.

Classification of occupation

Dissatisfaction with the Registrar General's classification led to the development of additional occupational schemas. The perceived lack of relationship between the measure of social class and groupings based on economic circumstances led to the development of a socio-economic scale which grouped individuals into 17 socio-economic groups (SEG classification). This scale was used by the Government in addition to RG Social Classes I–V from 1951. The analysis of the 1991 census provided information on both social class and on socio-economic group, which allowed consideration of the degree to which the scales diverged. Differences in classifying employers, managers and clerical workers illustrated the disadvantages of the Registrar General's scale. A further classification of occupations, the detailed Classification of Occupations and Directory of Occupational Titles (CODOT) was used by the Department of Employment in the 1960s and 1970s, but as it was felt that the combination of two Government departmental schemes was not helpful, it was agreed that there should be one Government classification of occupations from 1991 onwards. The Standard Occupational Classification (SOC) has been developed and from 2001 all national statistics data sources which collect occupational information will transfer to the updated SOC published in 2000. The classification depends on the type of work and skills required to perform the job (Office for National Statistics 2001a). Classifications of occupations, however, do not easily replace classifications of social class. In the 1990s the research community participated in an Office of Population Census and Surveys (OPCS) (now Office for National Statistics (ONS)) initiated debate concerning measures of social class. The Economic and Social Research Council (ESRC) was invited to propose a replacement scheme (Rose and O'Reilly 1997, 1998).

A major criticism of the Registrar General's social class scheme was that, in being based on occupation it ignored the relational aspects of class and was not based on any underlying theory about class formation. As Chapter One in this volume identifies, the two main class theorists were Weber, who saw classes as formed in markets, through people selling their labour, and Marx, who saw classes as formed through relationships — the relationships of employment or of control. Sociologists had developed alternative class schemes to the Registrar General's, based on employment relations as well as employment status. The three main schemes in use were Goldthorpe's, used in major studies of social mobility (Goldthorpe and Hope 1974, Goldthorpe 1980); Wright's, whose scheme is derived from explicitly Marxist principles (Wright 1979, 1985, 1997); and the Cambridge scheme (used in the Health Survey for England), which attempted to position individuals along a continuum based on evaluating own and others' positions (Stewart *et al.* 1980, Prandy 1990). As such the Cambridge scheme relies on subjective assessments of position and is similar in approach to the gradational Registrar General's classification.

Researchers' interest in the relational aspects of social structure has led to the adoption of Goldthorpe's scheme as the basis of the class scheme now adopted by the Office for National Statistics. This new classification still relies on occupation (and hence could not be used until the SOC was published) and will be used in Office for National Statistics data sources from 2001. It replaces the Registrar General's classification of social class and the 17 socio-economic groups (SEG). The classification ranks occupations according to work relationships of responsibility and autonomy as well as type of work.

National Statistics Socio-Economic Classification (NS-SEC)

1 Higher managerial and professional occupations
   1.1 Large employers and higher managerial occupations
   1.2 Higher professional occupations
2 Lower managerial and professional occupations
3 Intermediate occupations
4 Small employers and own-account workers
5 Lower supervisory and technical occupations
6 Semi-routine occupations
7 Routine occupations
8 Never worked and long-term unemployed

Under Goldthorpe's scheme, Classes 1 and 2 are grouped as 'service class'; 3, 4 and 5 as 'intermediate class', and 6 and 7 as 'working class'. Class 8 is regularly described as the 'underclass'. Readers will be interested to note that a report in *The Guardian* at the time the ESRC report to the ONS was first published notes that 'the chief novelty is in moving nurses up one class as "associate professionals", apparently because nursing is due to become all-graduate' (*The Guardian* 1997). The assumption is that graduate roles involve greater use of knowledge, analytical judgment, planning and organisational skills and greater exercise of responsibility and autonomy. These factors, together with physical, mental and emotional effort and working conditions are being proposed as contributing to the 16 scoring factors to be used in the job evaluation scheme which is likely to underpin the modernisation of the pay system for all NHS staff in the United Kingdom (Waters 2002).

The advertising industry standard

Government and social researchers are not alone in seeking to explore the relationship between position in the economic structure and other activities. The advertising industry is particularly interested in understanding how we spend our money. For the purpose of market research, the advertising industry uses a classification on the basis of occupation: A, B, C1, C2, D and E. This system is similar to the Registrar General's classification, and hence has similar strengths and weaknesses, with the rationale for the borders between C1 and C2 being particularly unclear.

Middle class and working class

None of the above measures necessarily reflects individuals' views about their own position in the class structure. Amongst subjective definitions, the terms most frequently used for self description continue to be 'middle class' and 'working class' and research comparing the distribution of the population using objective measures with people's self perception shows considerable discrepancy. Kirby (1999) provides a useful summary, drawing on the work of Hadfield and Skipworth (1994):

> Using the manual/non-manual dividing line as the basis for classifica-
> tion, the 1991 census revealed that the British population (or at least
> the economically active part of it) was composed of 56 per cent middle
> class and 42 per cent working class. However the MORI poll found in

1989 that 30 per cent of people described themselves as middle class and 67 per cent described themselves as working class. (Kirby *op. cit.*: 21)

Classifying individuals and households

There has been considerable criticism of class schemes that assign individuals to a class on the basis of the occupation of the male head of household, a conventional approach adopted in the Registrar General's classification and in Goldthorpe's scheme (only women living alone were classified by their own occupation). This conventional approach has been criticised for denigrating women's occupational position, and for ignoring the schemes' gendered assumptions which assign women's work low status and do not differentiate between clerical roles in which women predominate. In addition, the view that members of a household share the same standard of living and style of life has been challenged. Goldthorpe has responded to these criticisms by arguing that his scheme illustrates and recognises women's history of discrimination (Goldthorpe 1984, Heath and Britten 1984, Stanworth 1984, Crompton 1989, 1996). Goldthorpe has adopted the stance whereby the class position of a household is taken from the 'dominant' occupation in material terms. The 'dominant' occupation can be held by a man or a woman. In the new national class scheme, the NS-SEC, the unit of analysis remains the household, with class position taken from the person selected as a 'reference' person for the family or household. The definition of the household reference person has been reviewed (Martin 1998) and from 2001 the Household Reference Person (HRP) has been defined as:

> the person responsible for owning or renting or who is otherwise responsible for the accommodation. In the case of joint householders, the person with the highest income takes precedence and becomes the HRP. Where incomes are equal, the older is taken as the HRP. This procedure increases the likelihood both that a female will be the HRP and that the HRP better characterises the household's social position. (Office for National Statistics 2001a: 29)

Although other schemes, such as Wright's, have taken the individual as the unit of class analysis, problems in classifying economically inactive children or housewives are still resolved through relying on another's position, leading to a 'derived' class location. Joint classifications may answer some criticisms but introduce problems of their own, including the fact that very differently composed dyads may be placed in the same class position. Graham (2000b) explains that recognising the limitations of class as a measure of difference in socio-economic position has led to other measures of socio-economic status being used in research. Studies in the ESRC Health Variations research programme have explored the relationship between health and education, income, housing tenure and car ownership (Macintyre *et al*. 1998, Benzeval *et al*. 2000).

Measures of social deprivation

Researchers seek ways of exploring the relationship between different aspects of material and social advantage and variations in health. The importance of doing this (explored in Chapter Three) stems from the recognition that the relational aspects as well as the material aspects of stratification affect health. Wilkinson's work has suggested that among countries characterised by increasing wealth, countries with narrower income differences tend to show longer average life expectancy (Wilkinson 1994, 1996b). This has led to a closer examination of factors which may be linked to perceptions of relative as opposed to absolute wealth or poverty, such as housing tenure and employment security or insecurity.

Townsend has developed an index for classifying areas in terms of socio-economic deprivation (Townsend *et al*. 1988b). The Townsend deprivation index combines four variables:

1 The percentage of private households containing economically active members who are unemployed
2 The percentage of private households with more than one person per room
3 The percentage of private households which do not possess a car
4 The percentage of private households not owner occupiers.

As Blane *et al*. (1996c) explain, variables 1 and 2 are included as direct measures of deprivation due to unemployment and overcrowding. Variable 3 'is included as a surrogate for current income' (*ibid.*: 175) and variable 4 acts as a measure of wealth. The Townsend index was first used, based on census data, in a study of health variations in Northern England (Townsend *et al.* 1988b) and analyses were repeated using 1991 census data (Phillimore *et al.* 1994). The index has been shown to be a powerful predictor of variations in health.

The Carstairs deprivation index has also been constructed from four census variables, but these refer to individuals rather than households (Carstairs 1981, Carstairs and Morris 1989). The overcrowding and car ownership measures are similar to Townsend's but the unemployment variable refers only to the proportion of unemployed men and the housing tenure variable is replaced by percentage of individuals in the Registrar General's social classes IV and V. Again, this index has been widely used in studies of health inequalities (Carstairs and Morris 1991, McLoone and Boddy 1994).

As Chapter Three explains, the effects of education have also been explored in studies of the relationship between deprivation, affluence and health.

Sources of data and measures of class and inequality: developing knowledge about inequality and health

Our understanding of the effect of social class and deprivation on health has been greatly enhanced by the maturing of British cohorts of individuals who have been studied since birth. The success of early cohort studies in helping us to ask and answer questions about the effect of life circumstances and experiences on health and wellbeing has led to the development of further cohort studies and regular national panel surveys to monitor the state of the nation's health. These datasets, alongside census data, provide the material for many of the studies referred to throughout this book and many others concerning health inequalities. The use of the same data sets to monitor health and monitor social conditions and behaviours within a population developed through the early British birth cohort studies. The first cohort study, now known as the National Survey of Health and Development, was established in 1946 as a result of an investigation to examine the availability and effectiveness of the antenatal and maternity services in Britain. As Medical Officers of Health from almost all areas cooperated in this survey, health visitors were used to collect data. The maternity services inquiry was based on interviews with all mothers who gave birth in one week in March 1946. Although it had not been intended to study the babies, the Population Investigation Committee decided to follow the children and the study has continued, funded (with some difficulty) through varied sources. Results of this cohort study played a significant part in debates about selectivity in education during the 1960s and are reported in a wide range of publications (such as Douglas 1967, Wadsworth 1991). A subsequent cohort study, known as the National Child Development Study, began as the Perinatal Mortality Survey, sponsored by the National Birthday Trust Fund. This survey was designed to examine the social and obstetric factors associated with stillbirth and death in early infancy among 17,000 children born in one week in March 1958 (Power *et al.* 1991). A third cohort survey, the 1970 British Cohort Study, also began as a birth survey. With both the 1958 and 1970 surveys, the scope of enquiry has widened with successive attempts to gather information. A new cohort survey, the ESRC Millennium Cohort Study began in May 2001, with the explicit aim of collecting data to try to understand the social conditions surrounding birth and early childhood, thus enhancing knowledge about the intricate links between social and biological aspects of human development. These three cohort studies are supported through the Centre for Longitudinal Studies at the Institute of Education, London University.

Additional cohort surveys include the Office for National Statistics Longitudinal Study which is a unique database linking census data and vital events for one per cent of the population of England and Wales. At each census since 1971 the same sample is linked together and life event data such as new births, deaths and cancer registrations are added to the database. This study is seen as an important source for targeting health care, for policy development and evaluation, and for lifecourse studies concerning social exclusion, health and family circumstances, migration and fertility. The Longitudinal Study was established to check whether the persistence of mortality differences between the Registrar General's social classes was an artefact of the method of measurement and data collection. The health inequalities observed through the Longitudinal Study confirmed that health inequalities continued to exist (Fox *et al.* 1985, Goldblatt 1990). The main cohort and other studies are listed below.

Key cohort studies and surveys

1946 Birth Cohort (The National Survey of Health Development)
A longitudinal survey of individuals born in one week in March 1946.

1958 British Birth Cohort (National Child Development Study NCDS)
www.cls.ioe.ac.uk/ncds/nhome.htm
A multidisciplinary longitudinal survey of individuals born between 3 and 9 March 1958 in England, Scotland and Wales, with information collected at birth and at ages 7, 11, 16, 23 and 33.

1970 British Birth Cohort Study (BCS70)
www.cls.ioe.ac.uk/bcs70/bhome.htm
A longitudinal study of individuals born in 1970 with information collected at birth and at the ages of 5, 10, 15, and 26.

ESRC Millennium Cohort
www.cls.ioe.ac.uk/Mcs/mcsmain.htm
A longitudinal study of 15,000 babies born in the UK over a 12 month period from 1 September 2000. The rationale for the study is to understand the social conditions surrounding birth and early childhood. The health and wellbeing of parents and infants will be studied in the context of data about family forms, education, health, employment and parenting.

ONS Longitudinal Study
www.statistics.gov.uk
A study based on a one per cent sample of those enumerated in England and Wales, begun in 1971, with data added from subsequent censuses and from vital registration records (birth, cancers, death).

Boyd Orr Cohort
A nationwide survey of diet and health conducted by the Rowett Research Institute between 1937 and 1939. Follow-up study conducted in 1997–98.

British Household Panel Survey (BHPS)
A national longitudinal survey of household members aged 16 and over interviewed annually.

Whitehall Studies
Longitudinal studies of British civil servants, begun in the 1960s. The first study was followed by Whitehall II and Whitehall III because of the significance of the early results.

Health and Lifestyle Survey
A survey carried out in 1984 in England, Scotland and Wales. Two thirds of the sample were re-interviewed in 1991.

Health Survey for England
An annual survey instituted in 1991 to monitor trends in the nation's health.

General Household Survey (GHS)
A survey of households in Britain, carried out annually from 1971.

Census
www.statistics.gov.uk
The census of the UK population is carried out every ten years. The 1991 census included questions on health status (limiting long-term illness) for the first time.

The disadvantage of the main national cohort studies is that the individuals in the earliest cohort are only in their 50s and hence illnesses of old age are still not easily studied in relation to the influence of social conditions and inequalities. An earlier survey conducted by the Rowett Research Institute, headed by Sir John Boyd Orr, listed above, has been 'rediscovered' by the Department of Social Medicine at Bristol University. The original survey was conducted between 1937 and 1939 and consisted of a nationwide survey of diet and health, recruiting families from 16 centres in Scotland and England (Gunnell *et al.* 1996). Members of the cohort have been traced and a further follow-up survey took place in 1997–98, thus allowing lifecourse influences on health in early old age to be explored (Gunnell *et al.* 1998, Berney *et al.* 2000).

A further highly significant series of studies of cohorts followed longitudinally are the Whitehall Studies, also listed above, named because the cohorts being followed are civil servants. Given their relatively homogeneous experience, living in a relatively affluent part of a relatively affluent country, working in office based stable jobs, it was not expected that there would be significant differences in health status and mortality rates amongst civil servants studied over time. The first Whitehall Study followed civil servants (all white males) for 25 years. The results indicated that those in the lower employment grades had higher mortality rates than those in the higher grades. The gradient showed that position in the hierarchy correlated strongly with mortality risk (Marmot and Shipley 1996). Subsequent Whitehall Studies explore the relationship between health and inequalities further and include women in the study (Marmot *et al.* 1991).

Additional sources of data about health and inequality come from routinely collected information such as birth, death and cancer registrations. International comparisons look at gross national product and life expectancy to consider the relationship between national wealth and health. International comparisons can provide some important insights into the possible effects of social factors on health, and studies of migrants over time have provided useful information which has made significant contributions to the study of causes of heart disease, for example. A study of heart disease and stroke amongst men of Japanese ancestry living in Japan, Hawaii and California, for instance, showed that the rate of heart disease was higher in California than in Hawaii and higher in Hawaii than in Japan, suggesting that environment and lifestyle affected disease rates (Marmot and Syme 1976).

It is the abundance of national data about class, inequalities and health that enables the British Government to identify trends concerning health inequalities (see Chapter Three) and to develop action plans to reduce health variations. Researchers over the past two decades have been particularly concerned to ensure their findings have an impact on policy. Michael Marmot, introducing an edited book prepared by researchers at the International Centre for Health and Society at University College, London in response to a request from the World Health Organisation (Marmot and Wilkinson 1999), explains this motivation:

> Those of us involved in research on social inequalities in health feel particularly vulnerable to the 'so what?' question. Time and again we have been confronted by the question of whether research on social inequalities in health has any practical application. The hard form of this argument asserts that there are no societies without social inequalities, hence the research has little relevance. (*ibid.*: 1)

As Chapter One explains, the view that social stratification is an inevitable feature of any society has a long history. Whereas functionalists saw stratification as developing from societal value consensus, Marxism saw class inequality as an inevitable feature of a capitalist society. The current Labour Government, however, has taken the view that health inequalities are neither inevitable nor acceptable.

The view that class inequalities in health may not be amenable to change was strengthened during the decades after the establishment of the National Health Service in Britain. It was expected that this system of providing health care on an equal basis to every citizen would lead to a reduction in the class differences in mortality. Blane *et al.* (1996b) suggest that reallocation of occupations (such as company directors) within the Registrar General's social class categories means that the 1951 decennial figures for mortality should be viewed with some caution. The publicly available figures for mortality and social class following the 1951 census, however, showed an inverse mortality gradient with the standardised mortality ratio for men aged 20–64 increasing gradually from SMR 86 for social class 1 to SMR 118 for social class 5 (Logan 1959). Blane *et al.* (*op. cit.*) suggest the apparent failure of free medical care to affect mortality differences led to an increased emphasis on research which explored the effect of behavioural changes on health. If policy changes did not make a difference, individual behaviour was seen to be an issue. An emphasis on individual factors was supported by a political ideology favoured by the Conservative Governments of 1979–97 that highlighted the importance of individual responsibility in matters of economics and private welfare.

Within sociology, as well as health policy, one approach to explanation is largely to ignore structural determinants and to concentrate on the importance of individual agency. Such an approach in sociology has emphasised the importance of collecting qualitative data about subjective experiences and views of health (see Chapter Three). Popay *et al.* (1998) have argued that the importance of qualitative data is often overlooked. Research into lay knowledge (in narrative form) 'could provide invaluable insights into the dynamic relationships between human agency and wider social structures that underpin inequalities in health' (*ibid.*: 76). Hence research into inequalities in health relies on both quantitative data from major surveys and qualitative data from small studies. Nursing literature is also contributing to these more subjective accounts of the experience of health and illness in the context of individuals' lives.

Public health and data sources

Before reviewing current significant developments in both research into and explanations for inequalities in health, and noting the importance of these developments for all health and social care professionals, it is helpful to review briefly the links between data sources and public health policy and practice. Local, national and international research studies have played an important role in identifying the need for public health measures (Baggott 2000). Edwin Chadwick's report on *The Sanitary Conditions of the Labouring Population of Great Britain* (Chadwick 1842) clarified the relationship between physical environment and disease and was a significant impetus to improving sanitation, a key public health measure. Snow's work on the East London cholera epidemic in 1854 played a significant role in establishing the value of epidemiology. Snow mapped reported cholera cases and was able to detect clustering around a particular source of water — the Broad Street pump — thus focussing attention on the importance of water as a carrier of disease (Snow 1936, Pelling 1978). Baggott describes William Farr, a statistician with a medical background as the 'driving force' (Baggott *op. cit.*: 20) of the Registrar General's office which was created in 1837. Farr used mortality rates of poorer areas to highlight the importance of improving the physical environment of cities.

The collective orientation involved in attention to the health of populations, however, has always been at odds with laissez faire principles in economic matters and an associated ethos of individual responsibility for health and wellbeing. The success of public health measures associated with improving sanitation has not necessarily been repeated through measures aimed at improving the environment. Laboratory sciences such as bacteriology have led to greater health gains. Developments in the control of infectious disease through successes in laboratory sciences such as bacteriology gave impetus to an approach to disease control through preventive medicine rather than public health measures. This emphasis on personal health grew throughout the 20th century, at times appearing to sideline interest in the health of the population. When the National Health Service did not appear to reduce inequalities, both policy and research interest focussed on the effect of behavioural changes on health. As Blane *et al.* (1996b) report, during the late 1970s studies were established which attempted to quantify the health gain resulting from behaviour changes. In the United States the Multiple Risk Factor Intervention Trial Research Group (1982) followed 361,662 high risk individuals through a behaviour change programme aimed at reducing smoking and obesity and increasing exercise. In Britain the first Whitehall Study also explored health damaging behaviours and mortality (Marmot *et al.* 1978). Both studies found that behaviour appeared to be hard to change and behaviour appeared to have less effect on health than had been predicted. Researchers and policy makers also realised that although some individuals may change behaviour, they 'would probably be quickly replaced by a new recruit to the health damaging behaviours' (Blane *et al.* 1996b: 6). Hence difficulties with the 'preventive medicine' approach to public health led policy makers and researchers to seek different approaches which combine an interest in individual behaviour and the influence of environment and social structure.

Baggott (2000) provides a succinct account of the role of public health practitioners (Medical Officers of Health) working in the National Health Service. In the early decades — the 1950s and 1960s — Medical Officers of Health increased expenditure on local health and social services. Social workers, however, thought medical control over social service development inappropriate and The Seebohm Committee (Department of Health and Social Security 1968), established to report on the organisation of personal social services, recommended the creation of unified local social services departments which were outside of the control of Medical Officers of Health (Webster 1996). At the same time, general practitioners (GPs) were playing an increasing role in family health services. 'Public health medicine was in effect caught in a pincer movement between the GPs and the Seebohm reforms, and its future looked bleak' (Baggott *op. cit.*: 46). Throughout the 1980s the influence of public health doctors, called community physicians at that time, declined still further alongside the growth of both hospital services and primary care. This was also the period of remarkable governmental indifference to health inequalities, exemplified by the Conservative Government's ignoring of *The Black Report*, originally published in 1980 (DHSS 1980) and the subsequent report by Margaret Whitehead, *The Health Divide*, published in 1987. Both reports were republished together by Penguin in 1988 (Townsend *et al.* 1988a). Baggott notes:

> Throughout the 1980s, the UK government, led by Margaret Thatcher, was vehemently opposed to any form of central health strategy, despite being out of step with international developments. The Thatcher government favoured prevention policies that were consistent with its ideological position — saving public money, promoting managerialism in public services and encouraging individual responsibility. (Baggott *op. cit.*: 52)

Scepticism about the power of individual responsibility to achieve population health gains and concern about health inequalities and public health, however, did not disappear. Public concern about AIDS, drug and alcohol abuse, smoking, food poisoning, BSE (bovine spongeiform encephalopathy) and pollution and environmental health, as well as the activities of pressure groups and researchers involved in international research through the World Health Organisation, led to increased pressure on the UK Government to take a renewed interest in public health and health inequalities (Marmot and Wilkinson 1999, Baggott *op. cit.*). This renewed interest was eventually exemplified by an ESRC research programme on health variations, which began in 1996, and the commissioning of an Independent Inquiry into Inequalities in Health, chaired by Sir Donald Acheson, which reported in 1998.

Social scientists attempt to provide empirical evidence and explanatory models that reduce the significance of ideological positions in determining health policy. Researchers at the International Centre for Health and Society, researchers involved in the ESRC programme and researchers responsible for the longitudinal studies referred to above have all made substantial contributions to bringing evidence to the attention of policy makers through publications, and through being members of, and submitting evidence to, The Independent Inquiry into Inequalities in Health. The recommendations of the Independent Inquiry are having a significant influence on current health policy and were based on a careful consideration of evidence concerning social determinants of health (Acheson 1998).

This careful consideration of accumulated evidence has led to important developments in approaches to understanding the relationship between social environment and individual health. Early assumptions were that inequalities in health derive from inequalities in health care and access to health care, a view that has been modified in the light of persistent health inequalities since the development of the National Health Service. It was also thought that once treatments and preventive measures were available to combat infectious diseases, health inequalities would reduce. Evidence now shows that chronic conditions are also linked to social factors, which means that inequalities will remain as chronic illnesses increase amongst an ageing population (see Chapter Three). *The Black Report* posited four possible explanations for inequalities in health: artefact; natural and social selection; materialist or structuralist; cultural/behavioural. These are discussed in the next chapter. Macintyre (1997) argues that these four categories of explanation led to polarised debate concerning the relevance of individual psychosocial factors or material factors.

The available data from the sources outlined here, however, have led to new lines of enquiry into the links between social environment and individual health. Researchers now adopt less polarised views. The preface to Blane *et al.*'s volume *Health and Social Organisation: Towards a Health Policy for the 21st Century* notes:

> Research has pointed to the salience of the social and physical environment in which people work: to income, education, the organisation of work, to family functioning and people's psychosocial wellbeing as important determinants of health. Population health is predicated on widely shared economic prosperity, on the development of a supportive community life and on investment in people. (Blane *et al.* 1996a: xv)

Relevance for nurses and all health and social care professionals

This book explores and explains the relevance of research and theories about social determinants of health. Inequalities and health matter to nurses because nurses have played varied roles in health research and health policy as well as health care practice. They have played roles in the past in strategies to reduce inequalities and continue to do so. Chapters Eight and Ten explore the roles of district nurses and health visitors in health improvement. Nurses have also been part of the data collection involved in research, particularly major longitudinal studies and national surveys. Sometimes this role has been unpaid and unacknowledged, seen as a normal part of the job. Now nurses are recruited to research roles through national adverts. They remain the data collectors for the Health Survey for England because of their range of skills. Nurses also experience health inequalities personally. Their work environment can be stressful and their behavioural responses to stress can bring health risks. Nurses are amongst the occupational groups with higher than average rates of smoking and stress (Royal College of Nursing 2002).

Nurses are part of other people's experience of health inequalities, sometimes negatively through providing inappropriate, ineffective or inadequate care, often through no fault of their own but through a deficiency in service provision. Nurses have a privileged standpoint from which to understand the effects of social circumstances on an individual's health and have close experience of the cumulative impact of social circumstances on biological processes. Nurses' understandings of these processes may be limited and disabling or insightful and reassuring. A sputum pot can be a routine unpleasantness, a sign of self imposed individual degradation, or a significant mark of inequality through the effect of industrial disease. From a Marxist viewpoint, a sputum pot could represent the lung diseases suffered by coalminers; evidence of exploitative class relations. Ill health derives from the long term effects of working conditions which benefited the mine owners more than the workers (see Chapter Nine).

Nurses are also part of a health care system which has established targets in order to address inequalities in health. As well as participating in implementing these policy directives, nurses have considerable opportunities to develop new ways of working and new services and to participate in generating new knowledge through reflection and research. Blane *et al.* (1996a) identify key areas for further work: understanding the importance of income distribution; understanding the importance of work and working conditions; understanding the key role of education in quality of life; understanding the connections between the physical environment and health. To this list we could add: understanding the role of social support at individual and community level; understanding the links between psychosocial factors and biology; understanding the influence of social factors over the lifecourse, and understanding the significance of social exclusion for health. Chapters in this book explore these varied topics.

3 Inequalities in health: the effects of social class

Margaret Miers

Introduction

This chapter describes the history of health inequalities research in Britain and identifies variations in health which are related to socio-economic position. It explores explanations for the continued influence of inequalities in health between social classes. Other social variables including gender, ethnicity, age and geographical region are all related to health but these influences on life experience are not discussed in detail here. Gender and ethnicity are the subjects of other books in this series (Miers 2000, Culley and Dyson 2001). Geographical differences are themselves significantly linked to socio-economic differences and to labour market position, which are also linked to health; hence they are difficult to separate from social class differences. The importance of environment and communities is discussed in more detail in Chapter Ten.

Unlike many texts on health inequalities this chapter does not include a range of figures and tables documenting patterns of health and inequality. This is because such information rapidly becomes outdated and recent information can be accessed easily from a variety of websites as explained in the Introduction.

The Black Report and The Health Divide

The Black Report, published in 1980 (DHSS 1980), drew researchers' attention to inequalities in health in Britain. It was the report of the Working Group on Inequalities in Health set up in 1977 by the Labour Government, under the chairmanship of Sir Douglas Black. Patrick Jenkin, Secretary of State for Social Services in Margaret Thatcher's first Conservative Government, noted in his foreword to the report that 'it will come as a disappointment to many that over long periods since the inception of the NHS there is generally little sign of health inequalities in Britain actually diminishing and, in some cases, they may be increasing' (Townsend *et al.* 1988a: 31). This disappointment did not spur the Conservative Government to make the reduction of health inequalities a priority.

A further publication, by Margaret Whitehead and published by the Health Education Council in 1987, *The Health Divide: Inequalities in Health in the 1980s,* provided an update on inequalities during the 1980s. Interest in health inequalities generated by *The Black Report* had stimulated further research. The two reports were republished together by Penguin in 1988 (Townsend *et al. op. cit.*) and were extensively discussed by educators and researchers during the 1990s. The aim of *The Health Divide* was to draw together new evidence from 1981 census data and evidence from a range of new studies which aimed to measure the full spectrum of health and illness in addition to death and disease. The Health and Lifestyle Survey, in particular, provided important information through the mix of data collected. The survey was unusual in using physiological measurements such as blood pressure as well as interviews and measurements of income, education, housing and social class (Blaxter 1987). The Health Survey for England, initiated in 1991, has subsequently adopted this approach. Information about the Health Survey for England can be accessed through the Department of Health website (www.doh.gov.uk).

Mortality

The Black Report documented continued inequalities in mortality rates. From 1949 to 1972, death rates for adult men aged 15–64 were higher for the lower social classes than for social classes I and II. In 1970/72, for 68 out of 92 causes of death, the mortality ratios for classes IV and V were higher than for I and II. 'For only four causes were mortality ratios for I and II higher than IV and V: accidents to motor vehicle drivers, malignant neoplasm of the skin, malignant neoplasm of the brain and polyarteritis nodosa and allied conditions' (Townsend *et al. op. cit.*: 61; see also Office for Population

Censuses and Surveys (OPCS) 1978). Death rates amongst women showed a similar class gradient. *The Black Report* notes that 'throughout the 1960s maternal mortality fell by more than a third, but mortality among women in class V was still nearly double that of class I and II' (Townsend *et al. op. cit.*: 62). *The Health Divide* reported continued inequalities in adult death rates up until 1981, drawing on analyses of the OPCS Longitudinal Study. For the first time, mortality gradients for men could be compared even after retirement (Fox *et al.* 1985). 'Even in old age, men from occupational class V had more than 50 per cent higher death rates than those in occupational class I' (Townsend *et al. op. cit.*: 230). Evidence from the first Whitehall Study of 17,000 office based male civil servants also became available during the 1980s, showing that even within an occupational group, the lower the grade the higher the mortality for every cause of death except genito-urinary disease. The Whitehall Study showed a steeper gradient between the highest and the lowest grade than found in occupational class gradients based on national data (Rose and Marmot 1981, Marmot *et al.* 1984). A study of mortality from coronary heart disease in different ranks in the British Army also showed a steep gradient, with a sixfold difference between highest and lowest rank (Lynch and Oelman 1981). The significance of, and possible explanations for, these differences are explored more fully in Chapter Nine.

Infant mortality showed a similar gradient despite a rapid decline in the perinatal mortality rate between 1950 and 1973. In 1970–72 infant deaths in social class I were 12 per 1000 legitimate live births; in social class V, there were 32 deaths per 1000 legitimate live births (OPCS 1978). By 1984, *The Health Divide* reported that 'babies whose fathers had unskilled jobs ran approximately twice the risk of stillbirth and death under one year than babies whose fathers worked in the professions' (Townsend *et al. op. cit.*: 228). More recent mortality rates are reviewed later in this chapter.

Morbidity

Morbidity data were difficult to find at the time of *The Black Report* as the General Household Survey (GHS) had only been conducted since 1971. However GHS data did suggest that 'the average number of days lost through illness or accident among unskilled manual men was 4.5 times that among professional men in 1971 and 1972' (Townsend *et al. op. cit.*: 64). There also seemed to be a class gradient in self reporting of acute sickness, chronic sickness and GP consultations, with social classes I and II appearing to be healthier than classes IV and V. *The Health Divide* looked at GHS data from the 1976 survey and found that rates of longstanding illness rose with falling socio-economic status. Longstanding illness, however, was also related to smoking, education, marital status and overcrowding. Other studies (Hunt *et al.* 1985) used the Nottingham Health Profile to study self perceived health. This profile identifies the nature of health disturbance in more detail and has been used to look at the impact of health on daily lives. One survey found occupational class differences in self rated health for adults aged 20–44, with the lower groups reporting greater amounts of and more severe distress. Differences between classes were greater for men than for women, but after the age of 45 the class differences were small (*ibid.*).

The Health and Lifestyle Survey (Blaxter 1987) found that self report measures showed that those in lower social classes reported poorer health. The survey assessed the experience of illness through a list of 24 common symptoms. There was an inverse class gradient for a range of conditions including persistent cough and back trouble in men and headaches, palpitations, deafness and anxiety in women. *The Health Divide* reports that:

> when the prevalence of self-reported disease was assessed, lower social classes had higher rates of many common diseases like bronchitis, arthritis/rheumatism and varicose veins. With psychosocial health (ability to sleep well, concentrate, etc.), high rates of 'malaise' were declared by lower social classes, with the steepest gradients found in middle age in women and older ages in men. Physiological measures of fitness, like weight, blood pressure and lung function, showed the same trend. (Townsend *et al. op. cit.*: 234–5)

Health services and social class

Self report measures of ill health can be viewed with suspicion as a measure of morbidity. Their subjective nature makes comparisons difficult. Hence *The Black Report* also explored class differences in the availability and use of the Health Service. Measures relying on uptake of services, however, are also difficult to interpret. Use of services is likely to be affected by accessibility and the effectiveness of the service affected by quality. Hence rates of consultation are also seen as imperfect measures of the need for health care. Julian Tudor Hart, a general practitioner working in South Wales, identified one important criticism. He argued in 1971 that there was an 'inverse care law – the availability of good medical care varies inversely with the need for it in the population served' (Hart 1971). He noted that general practitioner (GP) services were better resourced in more middle class areas. Areas with highest mortality and morbidity such as the coal mining valleys of South Wales (in which he worked) were less attractive areas for professionals to live and had difficulties attracting staff. If services are not available, they cannot be used. Service use is an imprecise measure of need; nonetheless, research into service use has suggested ways in which social class influences health care.

Cartwright and O'Brien (1976), in a study of use of GP services, found that middle class patients were able to make better use of their consultation time than working class patients. Their study involved tape recording 92 consultations with elderly patients and interviews with patients and doctors. Their data suggested that middle class patients asked slightly more questions, gave more pieces of information and were more likely to feel the doctors would know them by name if they met them on the street. *The Health Divide* identified a range of studies published in the 1980s indicating class related factors which could affect use of services. Whitehouse (1985) found that transport difficulties to GP premises appeared to limit use of services, and Carmichael (1985) reported greater availability of dental services in more affluent areas of Newcastle-upon-Tyne. Pendleton and Bochner (1980) found that GPs volunteered more explanations to higher social class patients than to lower social class patients, Bucquet *et al.* (1985) found that social class I patients received more home visits than other social classes and Blaxter (1984) identified that classes I and II were more likely to be referred to specialist services than classes IV and V. Lower social classes made less use of preventive services such as dental or screening services (Jenkins *et al.* 1984, Marsh and Channing 1986). Nevertheless, data concerning consultations are difficult to interpret. Although data from the General Household Survey in the 1970s suggested that the lower the social class, the higher the rate of consultation with general practitioners, the picture fluctuated over the years. *The Health Divide* notes that two studies using the same data source concerning GP consultations arrived at different conclusions. Crombie (1984) looked at first consultations and repeat appointments and noted that social class V had more consultations for a given episode of illness. He suggested this was due to doctors compensating for lack of coping skills in the patients by giving more repeat appointments. Blaxter (1984), however, concluded that the higher consultation rates through repeat appointments were 'justified by the more severe nature of the illness experienced' (Townsend *et al. op. cit.*: 271).

Marsh and Channing (*op. cit.*) concentrated on looking at a sample of 'deprived' patients in one health practice and concluded that the deprived patients provided a 50 per cent higher 'morbidity load' to the service than their matched controls. This interest in noting the health consequences for particularly deprived sectors of the population has continued, notably through Phillimore, Beattie and Townsend's important study on widening health inequalities in northern England (Phillimore *et al.* 1994).

Explanations for inequalities in health

The significance of *The Black Report* lies not only in its collection of evidence relating to health inequalities, nor in the Conservative Secretary of State's rejection of its recommendations, but also in its exposition of possible explanations for continuing health inequalities and the subsequent productive debate, and theoretical and empirical developments. The report suggested four types of explanation for inequalities in health:

- artefact explanations
- theories of natural and social selection

- materialist or structuralist explanations
- cultural/behavioural explanations.

Blane *et al.* (1998: 80) claim that 'considerable scientific progress has been achieved by working within the *Black Report's* explanatory framework'.

Artefact

The artefact explanation suggested that:

> both health and class are artificial variables thrown up by attempts to measure social phenomena and the relationship between them may be of little causal significance. Accordingly, the failure of health inequalities to diminish ... is believed to be explained to a greater or lesser extent by the reduction in the proportion of the population in poorest occupational classes. (Townsend *et al. op. cit.*: 105)

Although this explanation received some support, and some close examination (Illsley 1986), the idea that differences derive from inadequate means of measurement has been largely refuted through the publication of new evidence from the OPCS Longitudinal Study and the Whitehall Studies (Marmot *et al.* 1984). The method of calculating mortality rates and social class used in the Registrar General's decennial supplements to the census relies on an analysis of the death certificates for the three years around each census (OPCS 1978). The numbers of deaths in each class are divided by the numbers in that class in the overall population, thus giving a class based mortality rate. The Longitudinal Study and the Whitehall Studies were established to provide information from more clearly defined populations over a period of time. Both these studies, based on identifiable populations, demonstrate clear occupational class gradients in mortality both across social classes and within class groupings.

Theories of natural and social selection

In this argument, it is postulated that men and women with poor health 'drift to the bottom rung of the Registrar General's occupational scale' (Townsend *et al. op. cit.*: 105).

This argument can be seen as linked to the functionalist account of stratification, which accepts the inevitability of stratification in any social group (see Chapter One). As Townsend *et al.* (*ibid.*: 105) suggest:

> The occupational class structure is seen as a filter or sorter of human beings and one of the major bases of selection is health, that is, physical strength, vigour or agility. It is inferred that the Registrar General's class I has the lowest rate of premature mortality because it is made up of the strongest and most robust men and women in the population. Class V by contrast contains the weakest and most frail people.

In a functionalist account, poor health brings low social worth. A lowering of social worth through deteriorating health would lead to 'drift' to lower occupational status.

Data presented in *The Health Divide* which support this view relate to social class and height. In a study of first time mothers in Aberdeen it was noted that taller women tended to move up the class hierarchy on marriage, while shorter women tended to move down (Illsley *op. cit.*). Similar findings emerged from the 1980 OPCS survey of heights and weights in Britain (Knight 1984). The National Survey of Health and Development 1946 birth cohort study has also shown that serious illness in childhood could lead to a fall in occupational class position by the time males were 26 (Wadsworth 1986). Further data from the 1958 National Child Development Study allow testing of the degree to which social mobility of children with long term ill health accounts for inequalities between classes in adulthood. The picture is not simple (Power *et al.* 1996, Kuh and Ben-Shlomo 1997, Marmot and Wadsworth 1997, Wadsworth and Kuh 1997). The effects of ill health in early life do not appear to affect individuals in the same way. Evidence from studies in Southampton showing that low birth weight babies were at risk of serious chronic disease in later life irrespective of social class (Barker 1992), however, has prompted considerable interest in trying to understand the relationship between health and social patterns over time. Blane *et al.* (1998: 91) note that 'evidence is accumulating that disease processes can have long antecedents', but although childhood health may be related to social mobility, social selection cannot explain all the social class health gradients. There remain significant health differences between socio-economic groups amongst young people whose social circumstances remained stable (Fogelman *et al.* 1987). This is a complex picture, with new data emerging as longitudinal cohorts develop.

Dissatisfaction with social selection as an explanation for inequalities in health, but continued interest in exploring the relationship between health and social circumstances over a lifetime, has led to the lifecourse approach to understanding health inequalities (see Chapter Nine).

Materialist and structuralist explanations

Explanations which emphasise the effects of the social and economic conditions under which people live and work highlight the role of the distribution of material resources within a social structure. *The Black Report* identifies separate lines of argument associated with explanations which can be grouped under a materialist/structuralist heading. The first emphasises the direct influence of poverty or low levels of economic resources. Marxist analysis can demonstrate the logic of this approach. In a capitalist society the inevitable economic exploitation of the workers in the pursuit of accumulation of capital on the part of the bourgeoisie would be accompanied by hazardous working conditions, poor housing conditions and low wages leading to impoverished diets for family members, including children. High rates of respiratory disease amongst men in the coal mining areas are an example of health inequalities being directly related to working conditions (Bloor 2002).

One argument against the continued significance of the intrinsic and exploitative nature of class relations under capitalism is the view that the capitalist mode of production has the capacity to raise productivity and improve living standards for all. The improvements in public health facilities and the scientific and medical advances which have contributed to the decline in mortality from infectious diseases can be cited as evidence for capitalism's and industrialisation's beneficial effect in relation to health and wellbeing. Major causes of mortality such as cancer have not necessarily been obviously linked to poverty. *The Black Report* noted that 'against this background the language of economic exploitation no longer seems to provide the appropriate epithet for describing "Life and Labour" in the last two decades of the twentieth century' (Townsend *et al. op. cit.*: 106).

An important argument against the view that economic exploitation is no longer a significant feature of contemporary society nor of social-structural effects on health and wellbeing of individuals is the argument that relative poverty has a negative effect on health. Even if absolute levels of poverty have reduced in a society, relative poverty persists and can still have negative health consequences. Even in an affluent society:

> those who are unable to fulfil the social and occupational obligations placed upon them by virtue of their limited resources, can properly be regarded as poor. They may also be relatively disadvantaged in relation to the risks of illness or accident or the factors positively promoting health. (Townsend *et al. op. cit.*: 107)

Since *The Black Report* considerable attention has been given to the significance of the relationship between income inequalities and health inequalities (see Chapter Eight). Debates about the importance of absolute or relative poverty continue (Wilkinson 1992, 1996a, Lynch *et al.* 2000). Advocates of the importance of relative income suggest that the psychosocial environment of an unequal society leads to ill health through stress. Advocates of the importance of absolute poverty suggest that it is progressive poverty of material circumstances that acts as the causal pathway to as well as the nurturing environment for ill health (Dorling *et al.* 2000).

Two further strands of argument concerning materialist/ structuralist factors affecting health concern economic trends. The effects of economic recession and unemployment on societal and individual health could be explored. *The Black Report* cites the work of Brenner (1977) as an example of an exploration of the health effects of economic instability. A separate argument suggests that economic growth can have negative implications for health, through the conditions associated with 'hazardous, punishing and physically stressful work' (Townsend *et al. op. cit.*: 110; see also Eyer 1977). Since publication of

The Black Report the health effects of unemployment and of the conditions of work have been considered in considerable depth (see Chapter Nine).

Cultural/behavioural explanations

In sociological terms, if materialist explanations emphasise the influence of social structure on our lives and health, the cultural/ behavioural explanations emphasise our own activity, our own agency. Cultural/behavioural explanations of inequalities in health focus on the individual's choice of lifestyle as the key factor in health and wellbeing. An individual's choice of lifestyle, however, may be influenced by the groups, including social classes, to which he or she feels a sense of belonging and affiliation. Nonetheless, within a cultural/behavioural explanation, it is the personal characteristics of individuals and their personal choices which are seen as key to healthy lifestyles. Evidence for this view lies in the fact that behaviours which can damage health, such as cigarette smoking, cut across classes. Changes in the nature of social structure and the possible decline of class (discussed in Chapter One) could mean that individuals are increasingly choosing their own ways of living. Lifestyle diversity could change patterns of mortality and morbidity. *The Health Divide* presented evidence about the most obvious health damaging behaviour. In 1984, whereas only 17 per cent of professional group men and 15 per cent of professional group women smoked, 49 per cent of men and 36 per cent of women in the unskilled manual category were smokers (Townsend *et al. op. cit.*: 291). Class trends in mortality from lung cancer and heart disease were similar. The highest income groups had the healthiest diets, measured by consumption of vegetables, fruit, brown bread, sugar and fats (Ministry of Agriculture, Fisheries and Food (MAFF) 1977, 1986). Higher social class groups also took more exercise than lower social classes, as measured through the General Household Survey. By the time *The Health Divide* was published, however, considerable debate prompted by *The Black Report* had led to significant theoretical and empirical developments in health inequalities research.

After *The Black Report* and *The Health Divide*

The Black Report had considerable impact on the research community despite the fact that the Conservative Governments of 1979–97 largely ignored its recommendations and focussed on behavioural explanations for inequalities in health, as evidenced by the *The Health of the Nation* targets that related primarily to individual behaviour change (DoH 1992). In Britain, despite a lack of governmental interest, research into inequalities in health continued throughout the 1980s. Bartley *et al.* (1998: 1) report that:

> those who continued to do research on social inequality in health were therefore under a heavy obligation of rigour in their work. It was a lonely time to be doing such work in many ways, but also a highly challenging one, in which all assumptions were questioned and sometimes tested to destruction.

During this period new data from birth cohort and longitudinal studies and the expansion of computing power confirmed the relationship between social circumstances and health. The debates around the four explanations laid out in *The Black Report* stimulated a search for a much more detailed understanding of the ways in which material/structural and behavioural/cultural factors interact to influence health and wellbeing. Macintyre (1997) called for a movement beyond binary opposition of explanations towards a 'more fine grained' (*ibid.*: 740) approach which allows a close examination of ways in which material and cultural factors influence mental and physical health. More detailed research has concentrated on a range of factors, with the importance of income inequalities, unemployment, transport, housing conditions, psychosocial environment at work, poverty and social exclusion, social support and cohesion, early life and lifecourse all receiving scrutiny (Bartley 1994, Marmot *et al.* 1997, Blane 1999, Macintyre *et al.* 2000). The research enterprise received considerable support through the UK Economic and Social Research Council's initiative to fund a programme of work, the Health Variations programme, established in 1996 (Graham 2000a).

It should be noted that concern to link explanations together has a long tradition in sociology. Social class research has always been concerned to link structure and agency, and whereas a Marxist approach to understanding social class and a Weberian emphasis on class as a grouping determined by market position would emphasise materialist/structural explanations, both these major theorists recognised the significance of subjective understandings of social position as influential in behaviour. Shared activities deriving from social circumstances could be seen as contributing to class consciousness in Marxist terms. Weber's identification of status groups as a separate dimension of stratification can help explain the significance of lifestyle choices within an unequal social structure. Recognising the significance of health related behaviours such as cigarette smoking for achieving and maintaining a desired social status within a peer group as a possible separate causal thread does not necessarily lead to a lack of interest in other causal threads (such as income level). New explanatory models in health inequalities research link not just structure and agency but also social, psychological and biological factors.

Interest in health inequalities was also stimulated through the activity of the European Region of the World Health Organisation (WHO), which published a common health strategy in 1985, with equity as a major theme and the reduction of inequities heading the list of targets to achieve by 2000 (WHO 1985). International and national interest and concern led to the Labour Government initiating, on taking office in 1997, an Independent Inquiry into Inequalities in Health chaired by Sir Donald Acheson, chairman of the International Centre for Health and Society at University College, London. The report of this inquiry was published in 1998 (Acheson 1998).

Health inequalities: evidence from the Independent Inquiry into Inequalities in Health and further reports

Evidence collected since the 1980s largely confirms the patterns identified by *The Black Report*. Class differences persist, and in some cases have widened.

Mortality

The Independent Inquiry into Inequalities in Health (Acheson *op. cit.*) identified the fact that since the early 1970s death rates have fallen for men and women across all social groups; however, the difference between rates for the highest social class and for the lowest group has increased. The increase in differences across social classes was apparent for coronary heart disease, stroke, lung cancer and suicides among men, and for respiratory disease and lung cancer among women, for all significant causes of death (*ibid.*). Between the late 1970s and the late 1980s the overall difference in death rates between social classes I/II and IV/V for men aged 35 to 64 rose from 53 per cent to 68 per cent. For women the differential increased from 50 to 55 per cent. Life expectancy for men in social classes I and II increased by two years over the same period, but the rise in life expectancy for social classes IV and V was 1.4 years. The differences between the top and bottom classes are considerable. Acheson's evidence showed that men in social class I have a life expectancy at birth of 75 years, whereas for men in social class V, life expectancy at birth is 70. The women's differential is smaller, at 80 years compared with 77 (*ibid.*: 13).

The year 2000 edition of *Social Inequalities* (Drever *et al.* 2000) calculated potential years of working life lost by weighting the number of deaths using the difference between the age at death and the age of state pension entitlement. The large numbers of deaths of younger men in unskilled occupations from accidents and violence means that for class V, some 87 years of working life are lost for every thousand men aged 20 to 64. The number of years of working life lost for class I is considerably lower at 27 years per thousand men in the same age range (*ibid.*: 20). Information from the 2001 census will allow further monitoring of these differences and trends in health inequalities.

Infant mortality rates are also still lower among babies born to parents in higher social classes. The Independent Inquiry reported that there was 'no evidence that the class differential in infant mortality has decreased' (Acheson *op. cit.*: 14); however Drever *et al.* (*op. cit.*) suggest that comparing the infant mortality rate for 1995–97 with that for 1974–76 shows a narrowing of the class gap, which may be continuing. The rate for the unskilled group in 1995–97 was eight per thousand live births, twice that for the professional group (four per thousand).

Data for 1999 reported in the *Health Inequalities National Targets* (DoH 2002b) show a social class V rate of only 1.7 times the social class I rate. In the mid 1970s the difference was greater, with 23 deaths per thousand for social class V and ten per thousand for social class I. Nevertheless the Government is not complacent and aims for a ten per cent reduction in the gap in mortality rates between manual groups and the population as a whole for children under one year old (*ibid.*: 7).

Morbidity

The Independent Inquiry reported an increase in self reported long standing illness (through the General Household Survey) since 1972, and substantial socio-economic differences. This is confirmed by the more recent report on social inequalities (Drever *et al. op. cit.*). In 1998, 33 per cent of General Household Survey respondents reported long standing illness, with 40 per cent of men aged 16–44 who are economically inactive, and a third of women, reporting such illness. In the 45–64 age group, nearly three quarters of men and three fifths of women who were economically inactive had a long standing health problem. Men and women who were working and those economically active but unemployed had lower rates of illness, with those in work reporting the lowest rates (*ibid.*). Unsurprisingly, men who are economically inactive have more consultations with a GP in a year than men in employment or economically active but unemployed. Among the employed and unemployed groups, women consult GPs more often than men.

Data from the Survey of Psychiatric Morbidity carried out between April 1993 and August 1994 show that women reported neurotic disorders such as anxiety, depression and phobias more frequently than men. Among women, these disorders were more common among women in social classes IV and V than among women in classes I and II. The rate for women in social class V was 60 per cent higher than that for women in social class I (Drever *et al. op. cit.*, Meltzer *et al.* 1995). Among men, but not women, there were marked class gradients for alcohol and drug dependency, with higher rates among lower social classes (Acheson *op. cit.*). Among children, a 1998 survey of the mental health of children and adolescents showed a strong relationship between family income and children's mental health, with 16 per cent of children aged 5–15 having an emotional, conduct or hyperkinetic disorder in households where the gross weekly income was under £200. In households where the income was £500 or more per week, six per cent of children had such a disorder. In families where the head of the household had never worked, 21 per cent of children had such a disorder, compared with the average rate of ten per cent. A class gradient was evident, with children from unskilled households three times as likely as those from professional households to have a mental health problem (Drever *et al. op. cit.*).

Other indicators of poor health reviewed by The Independent Inquiry and the 2000 edition of *Social Inequalities* include major accident rates, which, among men aged under 55, are higher in manual groups. Between the ages of 55 and 64, the non-manual classes have higher rates of major accidents. For women, there are no differences in accident rates except after the age of 75, when non-manual groups have higher rates. There is a marked class gradient in obesity among women, with higher rates in lower social classes. Women in manual classes also have higher rates of hypertension than women in social class I. Both these factors are risk factors for ill health, but there is no clear class difference among men (Acheson *op. cit.*).

Smoking ,

There has been a steady decline since 1974 in the proportions of men and women who smoke. By 1998 the proportion of men who smoke had dropped from half to about one quarter. The women's rate had fallen from 40 per cent to about a quarter. Throughout the period men and women in manual groups have been more likely to smoke than those in non-manual groups. For men the difference has remained at about 15 percentage points; for women the difference has increased slightly (Drever *et al. op. cit.*). Amongst teenagers, more girls are regular smokers than boys.

Diet

The 1998 National Food Survey, conducted by the Ministry of Agriculture, Fisheries and Food, showed that the amount of fresh fruit and vegetables eaten at home in Great Britain each week varied with the income of the head of the household. Drever *et al.* (*op. cit.*: 29) report that 'In households where there was at least one earner, those where the head of the household earned £640 or more per week ate twice as much fruit each as those where the head of the household earned less than £160 per week.' The consumption of vegetables showed a more complicated picture, with lower earning households eating more potatoes than higher earning households, but also eating more fresh green vegetables. The Independent Inquiry reported that people in lower socio-economic groups spend more on food rich in energy and high in fat and sugar 'which are cheaper per unit of energy than foods rich in protective nutrients, such as fruit and vegetables' (Acheson *op. cit.*: 65). The Inquiry argued that food poverty is experienced particularly by single mothers; it recommended a range of measures to improve the nutrition of young people including the provision of free fruit at school.

Exercise

The Independent Inquiry found no evidence of differences in levels of physical activity across classes amongst women. Amongst men, however, higher proportions in the manual classes have a high level of physical activity than those in the non-manual classes. Some of this difference derives from work related activity. It is men in non-manual occupations who have higher rates of leisure time physical activity (Colhoun and Prescott-Clarke 1996).

Socio-economic model of health

The Independent Inquiry adopts an explicitly socio-economic model of health. It identifies trends in socio-economic determinants of health. The determinants are seen as income distribution, education, employment, housing, homelessness, public safety and transport. The link between education and social class and education and health is discussed in Chapter Four of this volume. Overall, high levels of educational attainment are strongly linked to social class. Levels of attainment have increased significantly but there are significant geographical differences (Drever *et al. op. cit.*). There are also area differences in unemployment. The significance of employment and unemployment for health is discussed in Chapter Nine.

The importance of housing conditions in relation to health was closely researched during the 1990s. In England in the latter part of the 20th century there was a dramatic rise in the proportion of owner occupied dwellings (68 per cent of dwellings in 1997) and a decrease in the proportion of privately rented dwellings (ten per cent in 1997) but the condition of the housing stock varies considerably. The Independent Inquiry reported that 'in 1996 about 14 per cent of all households were living in poor conditions. About eight per cent of dwellings in England were unfit and about seven per cent of households were living in unfit dwellings' (Acheson *op. cit.*: 20). Homelessness increased steeply between 1982 and 1992 but has subsequently declined.

Macintyre and colleagues have conducted extensive research into the relationship between housing tenure and health through a study of adults in the West of Scotland. Through a questionnaire, the researchers found that home owners had significantly higher levels of 'mastery, self esteem and overall life satisfaction than renters' (Macintyre *et al.* 2000: 134). Owners also reported feeling more secure and more likely to report their health as being excellent or good and less likely to report long standing illness. In addition, owners reported fewer symptoms and had lower anxiety and depression scores. Renters were more likely to report occurrences within their neighbourhood which were perceived as stressors (for example vandalism, litter, speeding traffic, noise). Owners reported greater satisfaction with their neighbourhood overall. This research suggests that health is not simply associated with housing tenure through the links between housing tenure and income and social class. Overcrowding and dampness help explain the relationship between tenure and health (Ellaway and Macintyre 1998) but features of housing tenure may also be directly health promoting or damaging. The positive effect of ownership may work through psychological benefits deriving from a sense of ontological security promoted by a sense of protection, autonomy and prestige. Respondents were asked to respond to a Likert-type scale ('strongly agree' to 'strongly disagree') which included statements such as 'I feel I have privacy in my home' (protection), 'I can do what I want when I want in my home' (autonomy), and 'my home makes me feel I'm doing well in life' (Macintyre *et al. op. cit.*: 132, Kearns *et al.* 2000).

Public safety and public transport were included in the scope of the Independent Inquiry because improvements in both were seen as able to make a positive contribution to reducing inequalities in health. The arguments for this are looked at more thoroughly in Chapter Ten.

The importance of the relationship between income distribution and health inequalities is discussed more fully in Chapter Eight. Household income in real terms has risen considerably over the decades since 1960 but the increase in prosperity has not been equally shared. The proportion of people whose income was below half the average (median) income (the European Union definition of poverty) grew from ten per cent in 1961 to 20 per cent in 1991. By 1995 the proportion below half median income had fallen to 13 per cent but it has now risen to 15 per cent again (Drever *et al. op. cit.*: 36). Wilkinson has argued that the significance of income distribution, however, may lie not just in absolute levels of poverty. Wilkinson (1999) examined the relationship between population health and income within and across countries and suggested that 'More egalitarian societies, that is societies with smaller differences in income between rich and poor, tend to have better health and increased longevity' (*ibid.*: 259). Wilkinson argues that health is related less to material living standards than to position in society, or social status. Low social status in a hierarchical society has negative psychosocial effects and hierarchical societies have less supportive and more conflictual relationships. The logic of this argument seems to suggest that consciousness of class or status position remains significant in individual lives. Income inequalities lead to lower levels of social capital, largely through:

> feelings aroused by social comparisons to do with confidence, insecurity, and fears of inadequacy. Social hierarchy induces worries about possible incompetence and inadequacy, feelings of insecurity, and fears of inferiority. In contrast, the experience of friendship is primarily about the sense of being accepted and appreciated, and of having a positive, confidence-boosting, self-image reflected back. (*ibid.*: 262)

Wilkinson's work reflects a broader current emphasis within health inequalities research which is to study the significance of the subjective perceptions and experiences of inequality. Feelings and thoughts about social position and relative deprivation may bring stressors which, combined with material environment, diet, and addictive behaviours, have physiological effects which are health damaging. The evidence for Wilkinson's views, however, has been questioned by a range of researchers (for example Lynch *et al.* 2000, Muller 2002).

World Health Organisation initiatives

Many researchers giving evidence to the Independent Inquiry also contributed to a campaign to promote awareness, debate and action on the social determinants of health, led by the World Health Organisation Regional Office for Europe Centre for Urban Health. The researchers produced a booklet stating ten messages — 'the solid facts' (please see Box 3.1). Each message is supported by evidence and key sources, and the policy implications of the messages are identified (Wilkinson and Marmot 1998, www.who.dk/healthy-cities). These messages reflect awareness of the pathways that link the environment to individual physical and psychological health.

Some of the policy implications identified in the WHO booklet have become part of the policy of the Labour Government, particularly reducing the levels of educational failure; supporting families with young children; introducing pre-school programmes; increasing parents' knowledge of health and understanding of children's emotional needs; encouraging community activity; removing barriers to access to health care, social services and affordable housing; and improving conditions at work. The 1999 White Paper *Saving Lives: Our Healthier Nation* outlines the Government's public health strategy (see Chapter Ten).

The first main focus of Government policy in England, however, is children, as exemplified by the Sure Start programme (see Chapter Seven) and the national health inequality target to reduce by at least ten per cent the gap in mortality between manual groups and the population as a whole, starting with children. The second main focus is the reduction of area inequalities. In line with approaches adopted by other countries and proposed by the WHO, there is now a commitment to reducing by at least ten per cent by 2010 the gap between the quintile of areas with the lowest life expectancy at birth and the population as a whole. The lowest quintile health authority areas (prior to the 2002 reorganisation) had a life expectancy at birth of 73.3 years for men and 78.5 years for women, compared with average life expectancies of 75.4 (males) and 80.2 (females). These data relate to the years 1998–2000. The composition of the lowest quintile of health authority areas changes slightly but it is communities in the North of England which have the lowest life expectancy (DoH 2002b).

Box 3.1   Social determinants of health

- People's social and economic circumstances strongly affect their health throughout life, so health policy must be linked to the social and economic determinants of health
- Stress harms health
- The effects of early development last a lifetime; a good start in life means supporting mothers and young children
- Social exclusion creates misery and costs lives
- Stress in the workplace increases the risk of disease
- Job security increases health, wellbeing and job satisfaction
- Friendship, good social relations and strong supportive networks improve health at home, at work and in the community
- Individuals turn to alcohol, drugs and tobacco and suffer from their use, but use is influenced by the wider social setting
- Healthy food is a political issue
- Healthy transport means reducing driving and encouraging more walking and cycling, backed up by better public transport

Source: Wilkinson and Marmot (1998)

The pattern of deaths by social class across regions is significant. Whereas death rates for men in social class I do not differ across areas, men in social class V have higher death rates in the North than in the South, suggesting that although a professional person may be able to maintain health promoting conditions of life in any region, the characteristics of an area can have a negative effect on health (Drever *et al. op. cit.*). Since relative inequalities seem to have widespread health effects, action to improve health has to be targeted through area based and population based strategies. The Neighbourhood Renewal National Strategic Action Plan aims to support deprived areas; the Department of Health's National Service Frameworks (NSFs) for Coronary Heart Disease, Mental Health and Older People respectively, and the National Cancer Plan, are attempts to ensure inequalities in relation to key priorities are addressed.

Despite the Labour Government's claim to accept the importance of social, economic and environmental determinants of health, the reduction of income inequalities has not been a significant feature in its policy initiatives to address health inequalities. The Acheson Report recommends reduction of income inequalities. Hoskins (2001) has argued that is the key policy and that 'refusal to raise income tax on wealthy people has removed the most potent weapon the government has for tackling health inequalities' (*ibid.*: 29). Hoskins' own research into the benefits of raising the income level of deprived individuals and deprived areas, described in Chapter Eight, demonstrates the potential nurses have to make a significant difference to individuals' lives through raising income levels to promote health.

The significance of health inequalities research for nurses

The policy emphasis on reducing inequalities in health and on ensuring equal access to health care will be raising practising nurses' awareness of equality issues. Chapters Two and Three have given an overview of research into health inequalities over recent decades and alerted readers to the range of studies which provide significant data for professionals and policy makers to consider in developing policy and practice. For many nurses, the realities of health inequalities are part of daily life and work. I have argued elsewhere (Miers 2002a) that sound knowledge and understanding of concepts, explanatory frameworks and empirical evidence is necessary for care that is sensitive to gender differences and inequalities. Such knowledge and understanding of concepts, theories and evidence is also necessary for health care which is sensitive to socio-economic effects on health. The evidence on health inequalities suggests that the material conditions of people's lives and the social environment in which they live and work, including the societal and local status grading system, affect individuals' health, through the physical and psychosocial stressors that affect their bodies and their self esteem. Later chapters in this book explore relevant material and social processes and nurses' responses in their professional organisations and professional practice.

PART II

Nurses in the class structure

4 The class context of nursing

Elaine Denny

Introduction

The concept of nursing and social class is an under-researched area in the sociology of occupations. Although issues of class are subsumed under theories of power in much literature, it has been theories of gender that have dominated in the search to explain the position of nursing within the labour market. Class, however, has historically been a major factor in determining how nursing evolved, and was a preoccupation among many who sought to influence the way in which nursing was defined and constructed.

This chapter will consider 19th and early 20th century attempts to exclude the working classes from nursing, in order to define it as a professional occupation for ladies. Much of the impetus for change came from voluntary hospital and district nurses, but the movement was not uncontested, and the debates surrounding ideas of the nature of nursing will be discussed. Although these nurses were influential in terms of constituting an élite within nursing, numerically workhouse infirmary and asylum nurses dominated, and there was by the end of the 19th century a growing number of children's nurses. In each case their development is closely bound up with their relationship to this élite, and the extent to which it achieved its aims. These relationships will be considered, and the enduring legacy for nursing explained. Post Second World War developments in nursing will be analysed in order to explore class relationships that exist within current nursing, and to question the impact this has on the continuing development of the occupation. The symbiotic relationship of class and gender is acknowledged throughout. I will begin by describing social closure, which provides a useful analytical framework for the exploration of nursing in the class structure.

Social closure

The concept of closure was developed by Weber (1968) to describe strategies adopted by occupations to exclude outsiders and to create or maintain a monopoly, in order to protect market position in the face of competition. Economic reward is normally the impetus for closure, but status and prestige can also be powerful motivators to exclusionary tactics. The concept of closure is expanded by Parkin (1979: 45), to include the reaction of groups excluded by professional projects, which he calls 'the other side of the social closure equation'. This, he believes, links it more closely to Weber's contribution to stratification theory (see Chapter One in this volume). He describes the actions of both dominant and subservient occupations in claiming and defending an area of work.

Exclusion and demarcation describe the use of power in a downward direction by dominant occupations. Exclusionary tactics include the use of entry qualifications (credentials), legislation, or other means to restrict access and to define the boundaries of the occupation. They encompass a process of subordination, creating a group or stratum of inferiors, and are the dominant mode of closure. Demarcation is concerned with the creation of boundaries between occupations, and a dominant occupation will use this to control and regulate the work of a related subordinate occupation. Subordinate occupations may try to increase their status by attempts at usurpation, which is inclusion within the structure of the positions from which it is excluded. This is done by adopting the same values and characteristics as the dominant occupation, for example the creation of a similar means of self regulation.

Where an occupation seeks to gain inclusion to an occupational structure, while simultaneously excluding a group considered inferior from its own structures, this is labelled 'dual closure'. An occupational group may experience exploitation by exclusion from more dominant groups, while exploiting groups over which it is dominant. 'It is not, then, the social location of those who *initiate* collective action that determines whether the action is exploitative or not, but the location of those against whom it is directed' (Parkin *op. cit.*: 90, original emphasis). In essence, dominant or powerful groups primarily gain resources by means of exclusion, while for subordinate ones the main strategy is usurpation, with occasional exclusionary tactics.

Chua and Clegg (1990) propose closure theory as an appropriate analytical framework for examining nursing for the following reasons. Unlike functionalist theory it does not assume a shared normative order, or consensus. Unlike interactionist perspectives it does consider macro structures such as that of the state, which is crucial in the development of nursing. Unlike Marxist perspectives it acknowledges the pluralistic nature of class struggle, and does not rely solely on economic conflict based on the ownership of property.

Nineteenth century nursing reform

Traditional histories of nursing tend to focus on the type of woman who had carried out nursing work before the reforms of the 1860s, and the changes brought about by those reforms. The image of a coarse, disreputable woman giving way to the educated middle class lady, due largely to the influence of Florence Nightingale, was dominant at the time and still persists. This can be illustrated by an inaugural lecture, delivered on the opening of the school of nursing at St Bartholomew's Hospital in 1877, when Dyce Duckworth MD commented:

> Many years ago it was commoner far than now to meet with dishonest and drunken nurses ... Such wretched women are of course unfit for any responsibility, much more for such noble service as care of the afflicted ones of humanity, and they soon meet their doom in dismissal and degradation. (Duckworth 1877: 23)

The reality was that as nursing was unregulated, there was great diversity in standards. This diversity persisted, and as Maggs (1983) has shown, the majority of nurses continued to be drawn from the working classes following the reforms. There were, however, moves to change this and to make nursing an occupation predominantly of middle class women.

Why should nursing have been targeted in the middle of the 19th century for such changes? In order to answer this question we need to look at changes taking place within medicine, and changes within wider Victorian society. Nursing has always been defined and constructed by its relationship to medicine. By the middle of the 19th century, a period characterised by an increasingly capitalist mode of production, the medical profession was unifying into a single, high status occupation, with a large measure of occupational control. It was becoming more collegiate, and the voluntary hospitals, with their supply of powerless, mainly poor patients provided the ideal place for experimentation and research. Nursing work in hospitals had been largely domestic, but now doctors needed a worker on the wards who could observe changes in patients' condition, who could report this accurately, and who could unquestioningly follow instructions for treatments. In other words, an evolving medical profession needed a more educated, but also subservient assistant. Female nurses who had been schooled in Victorian ideals of discipline, obedience and chastity would be more malleable and less of a threat than expanding the recruitment of male dressers and clerks who might question the doctor's authority (Rafferty 1996). Around the same time many middle class women, either through necessity or choice, were seeking employment outside of the home. By the 1850s the 'problem' of surplus women (Worsnip 1990), women who were unsupported and yet not educated to earn their own living, could not be solved by the only occupations considered suitable for them — companion or governess. If nursing were reformed, and lost its association with domestic service, it would provide an alternative occupation for these women. There were also women who were rejecting the domesticity of Victorian middle class convention and seeking a role within the public sphere of work, yet finding the universities and many professions barred to them. So the needs of the medical profession coincided with the needs of a group of educated women. A reformed occupation of nursing could prove a suitable occupation for these women, who were already engaged in the management of the domestic situation, and in the control of servants.

The encouragement of middle class women into nursing was effected by redefining nursing work and tasks, and by creating a two tier system of training. Rafferty (*op. cit.*) argues that reform aimed at raising the calibre of nursing recruits was gradual, rather than radical. Indeed, Protestant Sisterhoods, such as St John's House, had been in the vanguard of providing good quality care, extending the high standards demanded by private patients into their hospital work with the poor as early as 1850. However, character was considered the major requirement for a nurse, and initial training schemes were designed to instill the correct moral attributes of obedience, deference, and subservience in trainees. Towards the end of the 19th century usurpationary tactics were attempted by the adoption of a more professional style of nurse training, based on science, and using the teaching of medical students as the model. The domestic nature of the work was now made scientific by the teaching of sanitary and hygiene laws (*ibid.*). If middle class women were to be attracted to nursing, it could not be seen as work which their own servants would carry out in the domestic sphere.

So a two tier training system differentiated between middle class and ordinary nurses. 'Ordinary' probationers would receive board and lodging, and a wage throughout training, whereas lady probationers (sometimes called pupils) would pay for their training and their board (Abel-Smith 1960). These ladies would on completion of their training be recommended for posts in other hospitals by the matron of their training school, and would expect to be promoted rapidly. As Chua and Clegg (*op. cit.*: 144) state, 'It was from this class that an élite cadre of sisters and matrons was formed that controlled nursing in the voluntary hospitals and workhouses both in London and the provinces.' Ethel Bedford-Fenwick, for example, became matron of St Bartholomew's Hospital in London at the age of 24. Ordinary probationers would become staff nurses in both the voluntary and Poor Law hospitals, but would not be expected to progress as far as ladies within the occupation.

Nightingale did not want nursing restricted to the middle and upper classes, and saw a role for the daughters of tradesmen and farmers. She nevertheless approved this division between the classes, viewing middle class women as possessing the leadership qualities necessary for higher posts. This two tier system reflected the middle class household, where the wife would have authority over servants, and would manage domestic arrangements. Carpenter (1977) points to the Victorian class structure as the basis of the hospital structure, with a division of labour between the sexes, and between women of different classes.

An example of the tension between the different classes within nursing can be observed from the correspondence of Mary Cadbury, who was an upper middle class woman, a Quaker and member of a family of drapers and chocolate makers. After training at the Nightingale School, St Thomas's Hospital, in 1873 she was sent to the Highgate Workhouse Infirmary, where she was required to stay for at least a year.

Mary did not like the Highgate Infirmary, especially the matron, Mrs Hill, who apparently disliked nurses who were 'ladies', as they only ever stayed for the minimum period, and then left for easier work. She did not make friends among the staff either. She confessed to Mrs Wardropper (Matron of St Thomas's) that the experience might put her off nursing forever, and subsequently wrote to her family:

> The patients are a much lower class than at St. T's, indeed I feel altogether as if I had come from aristocracy to democracy, nurse, patients and all and there is no one that I see to speak to. The only person I care to speak to now is Nurse East who came from St. Thomas's a month ago. I sit by her at dinner for we all dine together staff nurses and probationers. I find I don't like dining with such a lot of that class of people ... I take breakfast and supper in my own room. The bit of comfort I have is in the nice little probationer who has been doing nurse's duties [S]he is nice and humble and tells me everything in a nice way and I think she is a good little thing and doesn't set herself up a bit.[1]

Mary often referred to the social class of the nurses she worked with, and it was clear from her correspondence that she not only preferred 'ladies', but thought their work superior. She later wrote 'How different a lady does her work to a nurse probationer, she seems to put more conscience with it.'[2]

The workhouse infirmaries, like Highgate, continued to recruit their nurses from working women, and even from the inmates, middle class women who were drawn to nursing preferring the higher status and better working conditions of the voluntary hospitals.

This section has shown how in the mid 19th century the needs of a newly unified, high status medical profession coincided with the needs of a particular group of women.

For doctors a more educated nursing force provided a competent, yet subservient worker who could observe and report on a patient's condition. For middle class women reformed nursing, with its usurpationary strategy of redefining the domestic as scientific, provided an acceptable alternative, whether sought or not, to domesticity, yet one where the norms of the home were reproduced. Legitimacy for this hierarchical relationship lay within social class and gender relations. Within nursing divisions were also apparent, with a dual standard of training, and expectations of future status being based upon social class.

Philanthropy and professional 'ladies'

Not all middle class women wished to take up paid work, and philanthropic work with nursing associations provided an acceptable alternative. Freidson (1994) has differentiated between official, informal, subjective, and criminal labour and pointed to a hierarchical relationship between them. Official labour is paid work in the official economy, informal is legitimate but unregistered labour. Nursing work then, as now, took place within both economies. The subjective economy comprises those whose activities are not paid, but who do provide goods and service of value. The gain for the worker is symbolic, an occupation, or influence for example. Voluntary work is an important part of the subjective economy, and for many middle and upper class women in the 19th century provided the only acceptable alternative to a life of domesticity.

The model of paid working women being supervised by lady superintendents was common among district nursing associations of the 19th century. It was felt that working women would be more acceptable among the homes of the poor, where the associations were working, but that they should be supervised by someone from a higher class, with the moral authority to persuade the poor into a life more in keeping with middle class Victorian values. Legitimacy for the hierarchical position of paid and unpaid labour was the superior status afforded to women who did not have to earn a living.

The relationship between official and subjective labour within nursing may be illustrated by two nursing associations,

St John's House and the Ranyard Mission, in which it was in evidence, albeit in different ways. St John's House, which was founded in 1848 as a Protestant Sisterhood, was the first organisation to attempt to provide trained nurses for all classes of society, in hospitals and community. The organisation of labour was characterised by hierarchical divisions between official and subjective labour, and by a gender division of labour, with all females subordinate to a male warden. St John's admitted three types of women, whom it called 'inmates'. Probationers were literate young women who would be trained in public hospitals, and if satisfactory be accepted as nurses. They would pay an annual sum for board and uniform, and so would be drawn from women with some financial means. Nurses were drawn from probationers and from outside the institution, and nursed the sick in private homes and in hospitals. They were paid a salary. It was the Sisters who were expected to set a high moral and religious tone among the nurses, and who would visit, as opposed to nurse, the sick. These were women of independent means who contributed to the organisation, if resident, and who would set an example of religious piety and dutiful obedience to the lower class paid nurses. A demarcation can be observed between the official and the subjective economy, with the subjective labour of the Sisters possessing moral and supervisory authority. Nursing could be seen, then, as a vocation for the higher classes, but a job for working class women (Miers 2000).

The Ranyard Mission was an evangelical bible society which in 1868 began a nursing mission to the sick poor. Like St John's House, the Ranyard Mission demonstrates a hierarchical division between official and subjective labour, but whereas in St John's there was a demarcation of tasks, with more menial domestic tasks being the province of official labour, in the Ranyard Mission the subjective labour force of 'lady superintendents' was not involved with the actual tasks of the organisation at all. There was complete segregation of the official and subjective economies, with the subjective labour of lady superintendents being used in a supervisory capacity, and the tasks of the organisation being carried out by the waged labour of the Bible nurses. These were what Ranyard called 'native agents', respectable women from the same class as the person whom they would be nursing. They, it was felt, could more effectively influence the poor to adopt evangelical values of thrift, self reliance, and hard work.

Neither of these associations was concerned with the professionalisation of nursing, but later in the century many trained nurses came to view organisational structures such as St John's House or the Ranyard Mission as obstructing the achievement of professional status. One of these was Florence Lees who, with the approval of Florence Nightingale, argued that it was through district nursing (which in the 19th century was restricted to nursing the sick poor in the community) that the status of nursing could be raised, and become an attractive occupation for middle class women. Lees persuaded Nightingale of the necessity for district nursing to be the preserve of educated women, which in practice meant middle class women, and in 1874 Nightingale wrote 'On the whole it would seem to require a higher class of woman to be District Nurse than even to be Hospital Nurse.'[3] An indication of why Nightingale perceived the role of district nurse differently to that of the hospital nurse may be found in a letter to Lady Roseberry in 1888:

> The nursing of the sick poor at home is the highest branch of nursing, for the district nurse has no hospital helps but few. She must make the poor sick room a place where the sick poor can recover.
>
> She must first be a nurse but she must also nurse the room. That is an essential part of her duties — in cleanliness, in ventilation, in removing all sorts of foulness. And she must have the skilful tact and kindness to induce, to teach the friends how to do all this ... she must be a sanitary missionary, not an almsgiver.[4]

Lees became the first superintendent for the Metropolitan and National Nursing Association for Providing Trained Nurses for the Sick Poor (Metropolitan Association) which was established in 1878 to provide a trained nursing service in London. Under her influence the report of a sub-committee of the association, set up to inquire into the existing provision of district nursing, recommended that district nurses should have:

● a more complete and elaborate training
● a higher standard of general education, a more cultivated intelligence

● a superior social status, because she had more influence in making authority natural and in reconciling others to subordination and obedience.

Running through the report is Lees' conviction regarding the need to find suitable occupations for educated women (Baly 1987). Indeed, one of the objects of the association was 'to raise by all means in its power the standard of nursing and the social position of nurses'.[5] She wrote in her first quarterly report as Superintendent General:

> I give it as my unhesitating conviction that by limiting this work to well trained and well qualified gentlewomen, you will create such a class of nurse for the poor as no country has yet known or been able to produce.[6]

Unlike Ranyard and other district nursing associations which employed women from the 'superior servant class' (Liverpool) or 'respectable women' (Stratford-upon-Avon and Derbyshire) Lees held that it was only middle and upper class women who could influence the lives of the poor.

As with hospital nursing it was education, using a syllabus based on medical education, that was to be used to encourage middle class women into district nursing. Training would also be longer than that hitherto given to district nurses. Education would improve the social standing of the occupation, and it could also be utilised to exclude those women of the servant class who had traditionally gone into nursing. Educated women who had undertaken training could not, however, be expected to be supervised by the untrained, even from the same or a higher class, and Lees strongly resisted the use of lady superintendents.

In summary, a dual closure strategy was attempted by the use of usurpationary tactics aimed at using a medical model of education in order to raise the status of district nursing, while exerting exclusionary pressure to deny entry to working class women. These tactics were however not sufficient to make district nursing a profession for middle class women, as the Metropolitan Association could not impose its mode or length of training on other associations, nor could it prohibit untrained handywomen or minimally trained cottage nurses from practising. In essence their aims were hampered by the fact that they could not claim a monopoly over this segment of the labour market.

Nurse registration

By the late 19th century some nurses were looking to registration, a usurpationary strategy, in order to raise the status of the occupation. Only nurses entered on a register controlled by the occupation itself would be entitled to work as nurses. Witz (1992) has argued that previous writers have concentrated on the class elements of the registration debate, to the exclusion of the notion of registration as a female professional project. Nevertheless, part of the rationale for self government of nursing was to restrict entry to nursing to educated gentlewomen, ridding the occupation of the working class women whom registrationists, in common with Lees, felt hindered the professionalisation of nursing. Dingwall *et al.* (1988: 75) encapsulate the social class argument surrounding nurse registration:

> Was nursing to be a 'new profession for women' with a graduate entry and parity of esteem with medicine? Or was it essentially a refined form of domestic service, drawing on the considerable skills of many servants but assigned a clearly subordinate place in the hospital? Was 'proper work for nurses' the management of servants or carrying out the hands on services themselves?

It was a debate between those like Nightingale who perceived nursing as a vocation, with 'character' as the primary requirement, and those such as Bedford-Fenwick who wanted to develop an autonomous profession.

Self government of nursing was to be based around a one portal entry system to be accomplished by centralised control over the curriculum, the nature and duration of nurse education, and registration. Credentialism and registration together formed a usurpationary tactic; examinable competence and financial barriers (charging for examinations and registration) constituted exclusionary strategies. Many writers dismiss the battle for registration as being about snobbery, and keeping working class nurses out, rather than being about self regulation. Social class was a feature of the registration debate, but it was not the only issue that divided the protagonists. As Witz (*op. cit.*) points out, snobbery was a feature of both sides. Pro-registrationists wanted a middle class profession which would have the status for its members to enter into individual contractual relationships with clients in a similar way to doctors. Anti-registrationists saw a place for all classes of respectable women in nursing, but sought to restrict leadership roles to middle class, voluntary hospital trained general nurses.

Before the First World War private duty nurses constituted around 70 per cent of all nurses. Many of these were employed by the voluntary hospitals, or agencies, which contracted them to private homes, and set the fees and conditions of service. The private duty nurse was considered a superior servant, but one who was expected to know how to behave in an appropriate manner in middle and upper class homes. It was these private duty nurses that registrationists viewed as potentially analogous to doctors. Registration would lead to autonomy through individual contractual relationships between private duty nurses and clients, which would break the power of the voluntary hospitals, and the agencies. Registered nurses would have the legitimacy to control their own fees and conditions of service (Rafferty *op. cit.*). It was this that formed the social class basis of the registration debate, as only educated middle class women were perceived as having the ability to challenge the power of the voluntary hospitals in making contractual arrangements with middle and upper class patients.

In summary, restricting entry into nursing to educated women by the use of credentialist tactics was an aim of pro-registrationists. It was a form of social closure against the 'old' type of nurse, the working woman who had always worked on hospital wards and in the community. Usurpationary strategies sought to emulate the medical profession's autonomy in entering into individual contractual relations with patients. Paradoxically, as Rafferty (1995) points out, this autonomy was already enjoyed by the handywoman class of nurse that the pro-registrationists sought to exclude. The dual closure strategy of pro-registrationists failed in its aims, in that although registration was introduced in 1919, nursing failed to gain autonomy or control of entry to the occupation. The General Nursing Council (GNC) set up in 1919 to certify nurses was a body with few powers (Witz *op. cit.*).

Other nursing specialisms

Despite the relatively small numbers, voluntary hospital nursing was looked upon as the model to emulate, not necessarily by nurses in other forms of institution but certainly by their employers. This was increasingly the case during the years before the introduction of the NHS, when psychiatric, mental handicap, and children's nurses found that their qualifications were perceived as inferior to that of State Registered Nurse (SRN).

Psychiatric nursing suffered from the legacy of its 19th century associations with custody and constraint. Nolan (1995) states that Nightingale regarded asylum nurses as on a par with the lowest domestic servant, and gave them no recognition in her reforms. Ethel Bedford-Fenwick did not regard them as real nurses at all but as part of the penal system. Indeed they were known as 'attendants' before this term gave way to 'nurse' towards the end of the century. This antipathy was based on class and gender. Being mainly male they were viewed as a threat by those who were trying to create a wholly female occupation. As men who would regularly leave the wards in spring for agricultural work, they were seen as equivalent to labourers. This was compounded by their training of inmates in agricultural and similar skills. Many asylum nurses belonged to trade unions, with the National Asylum Workers Union being founded in 1910, which for the élite of general nursing further demonstrated their association with the working classes, and made them potential troublemakers. Asylum nurses were also tainted by the stigma and low status attached to their client group — the insane. At a time when general nursing was attempting to become scientific with its redefinition of the domestic as concerned with sanitary and hygiene laws, the asylum's association with custody and restraint could have hampered this professionalising strategy. Asylum nurses were, however, the intermediary between medical staff and patient (Nolan 1991), and as such were influential in the treatment of patients to an extent that general nurses were not. They also had a national training scheme from 1891, which was not achieved within general nursing until after the Registration Act of 1919.

In order to ally themselves to prestigious scientific medicine, psychiatrists attempted to redefine mental illness as analogous to physical illness, as having an organic base. The general trained nurse was perceived as practising a model of nursing more suited to this new definition. Middle class female nurses were seen as superior to working class men, and more likely to aid the status of psychiatry. So general trained, female nurses were increasingly employed as asylum matrons, bringing with them the values of discipline and obedience internalised during a voluntary hospital training.

Closely bound up with asylum nursing was care of what were then described as imbeciles or mental defectives. This became separate from mental health following the 1913 Mental Deficiency Act which differentiated between what we now know as mental health problems and learning disability. The ensuing institutionalisation and segregation of mental defectives was the result both of eugenic control, and of a realisation that they were not, as previously thought, uneducable. The legacy is therefore one of working class attendants concerned with custody and control.

Mental deficiency nursing became a separate part of the mental nurses supplementary register in 1919, but the recognition of this work as nursing did not guarantee acceptance, as the long term care and education which were the basis of their work did not fit the image of scientific nursing involved in cure on which the identity of general nursing was based (Mitchell 2000). The work remained low status for many years, until the closure of the large institutions.

Children's nurses were also viewed as inferior to general nurses, but in a less straightforward way. According to Lindsay (2000), during the period 1880–1930 the perception of children's nursing changed. Before this period it was associated with the domestic servant role of nanny and was therefore low status, the image being that of an elderly, illiterate servant. By the 1880s children's nurses were younger, better educated and expected to undertake formal training, often at their family's expense, which restricted entrance to the middle classes. Lindsay offers no explanation for this shift other than that nursing was becoming respectable. It is also possible that as lower class parents were often held responsible for their children's ill health, middle class nurses were deemed more appropriate to influence their behaviour. Despite this, pro-registrationists viewed children's nurses as uneducated, and susceptible to medical control (Dingwall *et al.* 1988). By the late 1920s there was much criticism in the medical press of children's trained nurses, who were unfavourably compared to general nurses. Even specialist children's hospitals preferred the general trained or dual trained nurse, and training purely in children's nursing largely died out (Lindsay *op. cit.*). So for much of the 20th century, paediatric training was an optional adjunct to general nursing, particularly for children's wards of general hospitals, where it was not uncommon for no specialist children's nurses to be employed.

Histories of all specialisms of nursing highlight the perceived superiority of the general trained nurse. It was the standard by which all other nursing was judged. SRN was the required qualification for promotion in asylums and children's hospitals as it was most closely allied to the medical model and to increasingly technological medicine. In this way it managed to rid itself of the association with lower class work in a way that the specialisms discussed did not. It was also viewed as the form of nursing likely to be undertaken by the middle class educated women who were expected to become matrons in all forms of institution. So class divisions were apparent within nursing, as well as between nursing and other occupations.

Registration in 1919 reinforced this hierarchy by the use of supplementary registers, but paradoxically it denied pro-registrationists the control over the specialisms that a one portal system of entry would have provided. The specialisms did not, however, view the supplementary registers in a negative light (Dingwall *et al. op. cit.*). Children's nurses hoped to gain status from an association with general nursing, although as can be deduced from the discussion above this hope was unfounded. The Medico-Psychological Association (MPA) which had an established examination and certificate expected to obtain delegated powers from the General Nursing Council, but again this was not forthcoming, although the MPA certificate remained the preferred qualification for both psychiatric and learning disability nurses until 1951.

One of the aims of Project 2000 nurse education (P2k) was to rid nursing of the status differential between its specialisms.

Students studying a common foundation programme would not only receive the same base for their nursing theory, but would learn about all disciplines of nursing. Dual qualification should no longer be the key to promotion. However, the impetus for P2k was general nursing, and there is anecdotal evidence that the courses were designed for general nurses, with the other disciplines of nursing relegated to branches. This is discussed further in the next chapter.

Nurse recruitment in the 20th century

Having established that the late 19th century saw a concerted effort by many nurses to establish nursing as a middle class profession, we can question whether the profile of the nurse did in fact alter. Maggs (1983) looked at nurse recruitment to four provincial hospitals between 1881 and 1921 to ascertain whether, by the turn of the century, the image of the nurse as a middle class woman was universal and an accurate picture. He found that many women had worked in nursing before taking up training, or in domestic or personal service (as companion or governess). He also found that many hospitals set entrance tests as the educational standards of applicants were so varied, but women from the middle classes could claim exemption as their education could be expected to be at an adequate level. While it might be expected that the taking of an entrance test or not would form a hierarchy within nursing, Maggs argues that those women who passed it could consider themselves as educationally equivalent, and by extension take on some of the prestige attached, to being middle class. This created a route to upward social mobility for educated working class women.

As has been noted, for some nurses class background seemed less important than certain characteristics — morality, obedience, truthfulness. This may have been expedient as the numbers of middle class nurses remained small, despite Bedford-Fenwick's assertion in 1905 that women had been drawn mainly from the servant class until Nightingale's reforms, following which a better class had entered, leading to higher standards of care for patients. Dingwall *et al.* (*op. cit.*), however, state that by the First World War the social background of nurses had not changed that much from the 1830s. Some well born women had become matrons or lady superintendents, but the majority of those calling themselves nurses were more working class. They were better educated than earlier nurses, due to compulsory education from 1870, but Maggs describes them as ordinary women who needed to earn a living.

During the war, however, nurses of the Voluntary Aid Detachment (VADs) upset the status quo, as many were from the upper classes. This was because as VADs were paid only in military hospitals, women with private means were far more likely to apply. For many women the work provided an escape from the middle class home, and, as in the 19th century, the fact that it was unpaid provided social acceptability (Roberts 1996). The result for professional nurses was that the lady nurses saw their exclusive position being downgraded by untrained women of their own class, whereas the ordinary nurses felt they would be further downgraded by yet more upper class women. It was, however, partly the influx of VADs during the war which provided the impetus for a registration bill in 1919.[7]

During the 1920s and 1930s recruitment to nursing was low and thought by some commentators to be because of competition from teaching, social work and other professions (Dingwall *et al. op. cit.*). But in 1939 the Athlone Committee demonstrated that competition was coming more from low level white collar work — that of clerical workers, shop assistants and typists (Abel-Smith *op. cit.*). Despite this it was advocated by the College of Nursing that payment during training be kept low to discourage all but those who had private means, perpetuating the recruitment problem, and demonstrating the persistence of the image of the 'lady' nurse. The College may have had an influence on the voluntary hospitals, but Barclay (1946) reports that between 1930 and 1939 local authorities increased salary rates, reduced hours and lifted restrictions on nurses' private time, and gave longer holidays and better accommodation in order to improve recruitment to municipal hospitals. This did not have the desired effect as other occupations, for example office work, gave women better conditions of service. Nor was recruitment increased by the abolition of minimum entry requirements into nursing in

1940 (a plank of registrationist strategy to exclude working class nurses), a move that was not reversed until 1962. Nursing it seems, with its disciplined and cloistered existence, was not an attractive career option for women of any class.

The situation was not however uniform across all types of hospital as voluntary hospitals had the pick of the available nurses 'drawn from the recognised finer social types, of greater culture and happier background' (Barclay *op. cit.*: 24). A careful selection of staffing was possible in voluntary hospitals even in times of nursing shortage, and some had waiting lists for training places even during acute shortages.

Barclay believed that the existence of medical training schools at voluntary hospitals gave the student nurse a 'wider variety of contacts, a higher social and professional level' (Barclay *op. cit.*: 28). While not explicitly saying that middle class women could find a suitable husband among the medical staff of voluntary hospitals the inference is apparent.

The difference in recruitment seen between the voluntary and municipal hospitals was evident following the inception of the NHS between teaching and district hospitals. MacGuire (1969) published a Ministry of Health funded bibliographic review on recruitment to and withdrawal from nurse training programmes in the United Kingdom. Like Barclay she found that recruits whose educational level was well above the minimum tended to be over-represented in schools of nursing attached to teaching hospitals, while those with the lowest academic attainment were mainly in non-teaching hospitals. Many teaching hospitals would set a minimum entry requirement of six 'O' levels as opposed to the GNC's two. However, she also found quite a range of educational attainment within training schools — some working class women with high educational attainment would not be willing to leave home to train, therefore trained in their local hospital, whereas some teaching hospitals might take a few women on the basis of a GNC test. The idea of leaving home as a factor in career choice is an interesting one. Abel-Smith (*op. cit.*) argued that nursing provided an opportunity to leave home, but MacGuire found that while the prospect of leaving home was a positive attraction for the better educated, it was a deterrent for girls with low educational attainment. In contrast to teaching hospitals, recruitment to non-teaching hospitals tended to be based on the immediate geographical locality, supplemented in many cases by overseas recruits. Recruitment to many district hospitals relied heavily on cadet courses, which would attract those leaving school with no qualifications who could sit an entrance test, or those with the minimum entry requirements.

The nurse shortage following the Second World War led to many hospitals employing unqualified nursing assistants to carry out the less skilled nursing tasks. This led to the introduction of the auxiliary nurse, and a second level of practical training, the enrolled nurse, for applicants with lower educational qualifications. Chua and Clegg (*op. cit.*) suggest that a denigration of the tasks that were delegated to these nurses helped to counter a potential proletarianisation of professional work. Although there is no agreed definition of 'nursing skill', registered nurses were said to perform the most skilled tasks, enrolled nurses less skilled, and nursing auxiliaries unskilled, non-nursing work, a demarcation of tasks which helped maintain the superior status of the registered nurse in all specialisms. Despite this, poor pay and working conditions continued to result in low recruitment, and the Platt Report of 1961 recommended improvements in both for learners, but this was again rejected by the nursing élite of the GNC who argued that it would attract the wrong sort of 'girl' into nursing. Like the élite of the 19th and the pro-registrationists of the early 20th century, the GNC was using financial barriers as an exclusionary strategy against working class entrants.

Conclusion

This chapter has considered the impact of social class on the development of the occupation of nursing. I have argued that the changing social structure of the mid 19th century was the impetus for the reform and reconstruction of nursing, although class cannot be disentangled from gender as a motivating factor. Credentialist tactics were employed in order to deny entry to working class women, or to restrict them to the lower grades of nursing. These tactics persisted, even during nursing shortages, in the teaching hospitals. At the same time usurpationary strategies were attempted in order to emulate the autonomy achieved by the medical profession, and to raise the status of nursing.

As stated above, nursing has always been defined and constructed by its relation to medicine. In a postmodern world that relationship has become more complex, and less monolithic. Mental health nurses increasingly see their work as complementary to psychiatry, rather than defined by it, and learning disability nurses view themselves as experts in a field where deinstitutionalisation has seen the decline of a specialist medical practitioner. These developments, among others, have seen a concomitant rise in the status of both groups within the nursing sphere. On the other hand, status within acute nursing has been to a large extent governed by an alliance with a high technology, medical model ethos and this has persisted. Areas such as intensive care or accident and emergency have higher status within nursing than care of the elderly, even though the art of nursing, the skills that could be said to make nursing unique, are more in evidence within the latter.

The concept of enhanced or expanded roles within nursing, such as nurse prescribing, nurse anaesthetist, or surgeon's assistant all add status by taking nurses further away from the caring role of nursing, and towards the curing role which has been a feature of clinical medicine. These roles all remove the nurse from the 'dirty work' of nursing, such as the management of bowel function, which Wolf (1996) argues has little prestige in society. Paradoxically these new roles also bring nursing further under the control of medicine. Rather than usurpation they are engaged in demarcatory tactics, with the medical profession defining the terms of nursing involvement, and, in the case of nurse prescribing, controlling accreditation.

The changes in all branches of nursing have been facilitated by the move from an apprentice style of nurse training in hospitals to the credentialism of nurse education, with accreditation by academic qualifications, in higher education. This will be a focus of the next chapter. As argued above, however, these developments have not necessarily given nurses autonomy or control over their occupation. Within the organisation of health work nurses remain, to a greater or lesser extent, constrained by class and gender relationships.

Notes

1 London Metropolitan Archive (LMA) HI/ST/NTS/Y/16/1 27.09.1874.
2 LMA H1/ST/NTS/Y16/1 06.08.1875.
3 LMA H1/ST/NC7/3 Suggestions for the improvement of nursing services of hospitals and on a method of training nurses for the sick poor 1874.
4 British Library add ms 45809 fol66.
5 LMA H1/ST/NCY/7a Objects of the Metropolitan Association.
6 LMA H1/ST/NC18/33/5 First quarterly report of the superintendent general 1875: 14.
7 For an interesting account of the VAD see Brittain V (1977) *Testament of Youth*. London, Virago.

5 Nursing, education and social class

Margaret Miers

Introduction

Several themes emerge from the previous chapter that will be explored further in this chapter and in the next section of this book. One is the relationship between social status and the views, values and activities of dominant social groups. Denny's account of nursing history in Chapter Four shows how views about the appropriate activities of 'ladies' had a significant influence on the structure and organisation of nursing. Higher class women adopted and retained leadership roles within the profession, partly because of assumptions about the moral superiority of dominant classes. Despite women's generally inferior social status to men, in nursing higher class women were accepted in leadership roles over working class men.

Divisions within nursing have always been linked to gender and to class. Education has also played a significant role. Changing views about gender roles, and particularly about the importance of education for women, have influenced men's and women's opportunities. As women gain access to an increasing range of professions, nursing struggles to retain its popularity amongst dominant social groups, particularly young, female, middle class entrants.

A second significant theme in Chapter Four which is explored more fully in the following chapters is the relationship between the values of society, governmental policies to promote change, the organisation of the health service, and nursing. Community nursing, for example, developed through a concern to influence the lives of the poor for the benefit of the health of the nation. But there were different ideas about effective processes of influence, leading, as Denny demonstrates, to different approaches to organising community nursing.

Chapter Ten reviews contemporary approaches to promoting public health and nurses' role in this process.

A third theme is the relationship between occupation, education and social class and the significance of social closure as a strategy to maintain social position. Not only does an occupation such as nursing change and develop in ways that reflect the values of society and the organisation of health care, but occupations are also affected by their market position in a class system. In Chapter Four, Denny explores the mechanisms used to preserve and enhance occupational position within a stratified society. Occupations which generally receive most rewards in terms of money and social status are those which are valued for their perceived high level of skill and for the perceived contribution they make to society. These skills and the manner in which they are acquired may be worth usurping. In adopting a model of education based on science, for example, Denny has suggested that nursing sought status through taking medicine as its model. Chapter Four also illustrates the importance of educational qualifications in validating activities and types of knowledge as well as in denigrating and subordinating those excluded from professional training. The assumed superiority of general nurse training and the importance of a general nursing qualification for leadership positions throughout much of the 20th century illustrates the strength of the link between qualifications and opportunities.

Whereas functionalist explanations saw status as deriving from value consensus, Weber (1945, 1968), Freidson (1970, 1994), Johnson (1972) and others have identified the role of power in maintaining professional status. Exclusionary strategies adopted to maintain occupational position have been self regulation, control over entry to the occupation and control over education and training. The nurse registration movement was both a battle for self regulation and an attempt to restrict entry into the profession. Educational qualifications have been an important means of securing social status and occupational mobility for women (Savage and Egerton 1997) and the nature and location of nurse education probably remains an important influence on nursing's position in a class structure. To gain an equivalent status position to teachers, managers, solicitors or doctors, nurses require an equivalent professional education. This chapter, therefore, considers the central importance of nurses' position in an educational hierarchy both for nurses' own perceptions of status and society's expectations of nursing as a profession. It concludes with a discussion of the significance of educational development for role development and for individual nurses.

Social class and education

A feature of the latter part of the 20th century was the increase in the importance of educational qualifications in securing employment. All approaches to understanding inequalities acknowledge the relationship between socio-economic inequalities and education. Higher educational qualifications and length of education are closely associated with middle class and professional jobs and with valued skills in society. The expansion of higher educational opportunities through the last thirty years of the 20th century accompanied the changing shape of the class structure in Britain. Kirby (1999) collates census data from the Office for National Statistics showing that the proportion of the population in social classes IV and V declined from 29 per cent in 1971 to 21 per cent in 1991. The proportion in social classes I and II has increased from 22 per cent in 1971 to 33 per cent in 1991. The growth in non-manual occupations, particularly service occupations, professional and managerial roles has been supported and accompanied by higher participation rates in post-compulsory education (Roberts 2001). Although expansion of educational opportunities may have been intended to improve opportunities for the children of manual workers, the middle class has benefited from policies to expand educational opportunities as much as the working class (Halsey *et al.* 1980, Roberts *op. cit.*). The expansion of higher education during the 1990s increased the proportion of middle class as well as working class children entering university. Middle class advantage seems to be preserved through, for example, access to private schools and hence to high levels of achievement in examinations which lead to access to top ranking universities. Degrees from top ranking universities continue to bring a form of 'cultural capital'

(Bourdieu 1986) largely unavailable to graduates from universities which were formerly polytechnics. Reay *et al.* (2001: 861) have shown how 'material constraints of travel and finance' restrict choices of higher education institution for working class students. Such students are more likely than middle class students to attend a university local to their home. Nevertheless, expansion of educational opportunities has led to some absolute mobility for the working class and for women (Savage and Egerton *op. cit.*).

Some of the expansion of higher education in the 20th century has been attributable to the movement of predominantly female professions into higher education. Teacher training moved into universities and polytechnics during the 1970s. Allied health professions followed during the 1980s and 1990s. Although nursing was slow to make this move, by the end of 1996, in Britain, all nurses and midwives were being educated in higher education, following a process of incorporation of Colleges of Health and Colleges of Nursing and Midwifery into universities or other higher education institutions. This incorporation process followed the Project 2000 (UKCC 1986) reforms in nurse education which unified nurse education by ending enrolled nurse training and introducing the common foundation programme to underpin specialist training in mental health, learning disabilities, adult and children's nursing. Project 2000 thus attempted (not necessarily with success) to reduce the divisions within the profession and to end the superiority of general nursing as a qualification perceived as necessary for other nursing branches. The late entry of nursing into higher education, however, should be considered in relation to both gender and class inequalities. The significance of late entry can be considered in relation to the advantages of education for individuals and social groups in terms of what Wadsworth (1996) terms 'health capital'.

Education and health

Educational qualifications are significant for an individual's life chances for several reasons. Qualifications lead to employment, status and income. Higher levels of education also lead to healthier lifestyles. There is a substantial gradient by education level in the odds of being a smoker, for example. Those with no educational qualifications are more than twice as likely to smoke than individuals educated to degree level (Jarvis and Wardle 1999). There is widespread evidence that individuals with low levels of education are least likely or slowest to respond to health education messages (Wadsworth *op. cit.*). Wadsworth's analyses of data from the 1946 birth cohort study (The National Survey of Health and Development) have identified the fact that:

> parental enthusiasm for education was found to be associated many years later, at age 43 years, with raised optimism about current and future work, achievements and opportunities, regardless of current social class in men, but in women comparable levels of optimism were found only among those in non-manual occupations. (*ibid.*: 157)

Benefits of higher educational attainment included 'greater involvement in arts, politics and sport, greater acceptance of new ideas, and higher enthusiasm for the education of offspring' (*ibid.*: 158) as well as likelihood of higher earnings. Education can contribute to health capital through the consequences of adequate income, feeling of security and purpose and access to ideas about health care. At a population level, Muller (2002) has argued, on the basis of cross sectional, multiple regression analysis of United States census statistics, that possession or lack of completed high school education was a more powerful predictor of differences in mortality than income inequality. It is unclear, however, whether low educational status affects health because of its negative influence on income or through feelings of deprivation associated with low relative position in the social hierarchy.

Class and classification in education: defining knowledge and skill

Higher levels of education have hitherto only been seen as necessary for a relatively restricted range of occupations and activities. Activities seen as requiring significant educational preparation are those perceived as having value at one point in time. The value placed on the activity, however, is not independent of judgments made about who carries out the activity, or where the activity takes place. Work carried out mainly by women has not been highly valued in the past and work that takes place in the private sphere of the home has been seen as less significant (even in sociology) than public service and paid employment outside the home (Oakley 1974, Abbott and Wallace 1990). Nurses' position in the labour market aligns with societal expectations of women, and with societal valuing of a range of activities nurses have undertaken, from cleaning, personal care, monitoring of treatment to the growing range of activities related to administering and prescribing treatment and planning and providing care and support. Hence, although nursing is seen as a profession it is not in the highest social group (see Chapter Two) and the knowledge and skills nurses need have not necessarily been seen as warranting lengthy educational support.

The education system works in alignment with the occupational system, supporting the development of knowledge and skills. In the past the education system has classified knowledge and skill (and therefore classified individuals) through shaping curricula and through restricting access to types of educational opportunities. Processes of selection of children into types of schools, such as the practice in the 1950s of selecting children for grammar schools through performance in tests at age 11, are obvious means of using educational classifications at a system level to support a social division of labour. Grammar school education emphasised intellectual development and academic knowledge relevant for the examinations ('A' levels) that controlled access to universities and to higher status jobs, including the legal and medical professions. Other secondary schools emphasised development for employment skills. In comprehensive schools, approaches to streaming pupils by ability could also contribute to supporting a class based division of labour (Willis 1977). Professional bodies have similarly controlled access to professional knowledge and expertise through controlling access to professional training. As Hugman (1991) has noted, power is linked to claims to knowledge and any profession will attempt to retain control over its own knowledge base. Nursing's attempts to develop its own knowledge base and to exert control over its own education have inevitably been constrained by discourses about gender and, as Denny has already made clear in the previous chapter, by class. The constraints of these discourses may explain nursing's tardiness in seeking a university based education.

Gender and curricula: implications for nursing

Educational opportunities become constrained through curriculum choices and decisions. In the past, offering girls and boys different opportunities to study cookery or metalwork were practices that sustained a gender division of labour. Victorian middle class emphasis on the importance of character and feminine accomplishments became linked to the perceived qualities of an educated woman through highlighting the study of literature and the arts. Girls' grammar school education, and subsequently choice of university degree during the 1950s and 1960s, emphasised the arts, reflecting a middle and upper class view of the educated woman as artistic, well read and intellectual. Such women did not need to earn their own living but would ensure that their children gained the appropriate intellectual and verbal skills necessary for middle class professional and managerial roles. Middleton (1987) has shown how streaming in schools restricted access to particular subjects and helped construct practical skills as separate from, and inferior to, intellectual ability. The restrictive nature of curricula for girls has been widely recognised and has now changed. Nevertheless, nursing has been affected by such restrictive practices, through an emphasis on nursing activities as women's work and the low status of caring within curricula. Skeggs (1997) has argued that caring courses have had the lowest status in subject rankings. In her study of women following caring courses in further education she noted that the women were aware of the distinctions made between different courses and of their own low status in the education hierarchy. As a result the young women came to give prominence to the value of their practical experience at the expense of their academic studies, in order to shape their own sense of achievement. Their sense of responsibility and respectability — their social status — derived from their responsibility for caring for others (*ibid.*). I have noted the relevance of Skeggs' work for nursing elsewhere (Miers 2000). I have also argued that the denigration of caring and practical skills within the education hierarchy has led to an anti-intellectualism within nursing which has justified denigrating the achievements of nurses with high academic qualifications. Bright girls have not necessarily been welcome in the profession (Miers 2002b). Nursing may have also contributed to its own low status by putting most stress on the practical and experiential nature of nursing knowledge and denigrating the intellectual and evidence based traditions of professional knowledge. Thompson and Watson (2001), however, have expressed concern that the wholesale move of nursing into higher education may have been premature. They bemoan the lack of support for scholarship in nursing and identify 'an anti-intellectual ethos pervading nursing' in which anything 'perceived to be intellectual is criticised as élitist ... curiosity, creativity and a passion for ideas seem to be out-moded' (*ibid.*: 1).

In nursing, the emphasis on the importance of practical experience does appear to have led to a resistance to participating in, and valuing, research. Hicks (1996, 1999) has shown how nurses' views may have an inhibiting effect on nursing's participation in research, essential to the development of nursing as a significant profession. In studies of nurses' assumptions about a range of qualities of hypothetical candidates for a nursing post, described as either a good researcher or a good clinician, Hicks found that the candidate rated as a good researcher was assumed to be more ambitious, a poorer communicator, less kind, stronger, more logical, more controlled, more confident, less popular, more ruthless, more rational and more analytical than the candidate described as a good clinician. Hicks (1996: 359) argues that:

> the results from this study suggest that if a nurse is described as a good researcher then the traits attributed to her are incompatible with those of a good clinician. Moreover, the converse also applies, in that a nurse who is a good clinician is assumed to possess characteristics which may not befit a good researcher.

In her later study Hicks (1999: 138) found that 'Male and female nurse raters construe men and researchers to be more ambitious and successful, yet less kind and compassionate.' She explores the implications of her findings in relation to traditional assumptions about the qualities of a good nurse, and the inextricable relationship between nursing and gender, and notes that 'to excel in nursing research it may be necessary to abandon some fundamental values on which nursing is founded' (*ibid.*: 130). Since men are not stereotypical nurses, Hicks suggests that if her results are generalisable, ' it is quite possible that unless some impact can be made on the collective stereotypes, female nurses will, for the foreseeable future, be confined to lower grade clinical roles, while male nurses will be eased into higher grade management and prestigious research roles' (*ibid.*: 138). Hicks' work has clear implications for women nurses but it is also illustrative of traditional perceptions of hierarchies of skill and class differences in valued attributes. The success of men in gaining nursing management roles in the latter part of the 20th century may be because men did not adopt the prevailing anti-intellectualism within nursing. However the attitudes of a minority (men) were not likely to have a significant impact on the culture of the profession.

Nursing's ambivalence towards research is also reflected in its ambivalence about degree level education. The profession did not necessarily welcome graduate nurses. Wright (1996) records that nurses from the first degree course established at Edinburgh University were shocked by their reception on qualifying. Superiors and colleagues were hostile to the graduates. As Sarah Witcher, a student on the first undergraduate degree programme noted, 'nursing wasn't something you did if you were academically minded' (*ibid.*: 17). Burke and Harris (2000), in a survey of 34 educational purchasers, found continued reservations about the need for a graduate nursing workforce as many nursing activities are not perceived as requiring graduate level skill. Nonetheless the purchasers agreed about graduate qualities which they saw as 'the ability to be reflective, to question practice and to be more sensitive to the needs of clients' (*ibid.*: 626). Nursing remains the only major health profession without graduate entry for all recruits. Allied health professions and midwifery now have degree level initial qualification.

Nursing, education and social class

Nursing's ambivalence about degree level and higher education in fact probably reflects the class origins of the majority of
nurses. The ambivalence can be seen as reflecting an accurate
understanding of the way in which the education system supported the class system in the United Kingdom, a class system
which did not give high status to the work nurses do. The
class based nature of higher education in Britain has been
strongly criticised and signs of continued élitism on the part of
leading universities is now regularly under attack. Current
educational policy, under the Labour Government since 1997,
is attempting to break down the class based élitism which has
been embedded in British education for many decades. The commitment to ensure change is exemplified by the Government's
target of 50 per cent participation in higher education by
2010 (Universities UK 2002). At the same time education
policy is also trying to develop high skill levels appropriate to
an economy which relies on specialist technical and knowledge
based skills. Britain's separation of academic and vocational
education has not necessarily supported a high skill economy.
Robertson (2002: 12) notes that similar economies such as
the United States of America, France and Germany:

> get it right in their different ways with an appropriate mix of high and
> intermediate level skills combining the academic and vocational,
> spread across a broad social space and across more differentiated
> institutions than in the UK.

Robertson (*ibid*.: 12) argues that the United Kingdom:

> lags behind these competitors in socially fair entry and meritocratic
> student progression. We are far from purging our national culture of
> class based attitudes towards the institutions, qualifications and prac-
> tices we define as valuable.

Strategies to promote inclusivity alongside high skill include
a coherent educational 'climbing frame' or 'skills escalator'
(DoH 2001c) which allows movement across and up vocational
and academic sectors. A structure of educational opportunities
of this nature must involve valuing a range of practical, technical, interpersonal and intellectual skills.

The class based nature of educational opportunities in
Britain is now seen as having a range of negative consequences,

including the rejection of intellectual ability and academic success by groups whose own skills have not been accorded high status. This is seen as having an inhibiting effect on participation rates in higher education. It is white working class males who have the lowest participation rate. Boys are falling behind girls in gaining educational qualifications at secondary school.

While such a class based educational system persisted, the separation of the majority of nurse education courses from higher education until the Project 2000 (UKCC *op. cit.*) reforms had many consequences for nursing. It ensured that nursing was not the choice of middle class women in the latter part of the 20th century despite nursing's relatively high status as a respectable profession for women. A complex mesh of factors sustained and supported this separation. These included discourses about women's role and discourses about education within nursing.

Discourses about women's role

Hicks' (1996, 1999) work confirms that it is difficult to make sense of different views within and about nursing without considering discourses about women's role and nursing's involvement in such discourses. Women's increased participation in higher education during the 1960s and 1970s was accompanied by a 'second wave' of feminism as an influential analysis of men and women's position in social structures. Feminism emphasised women's equal right to participate in public activities. Somerville (1997: 678) notes that the women's liberation movement in the 1960s identified women's inequalities in relation to men as a consequence of:

> interpersonal relations of power between men and women. Thus the struggle for women's liberation had to begin by fundamentally changing those institutions and practices which bind women into the private life, in particular the conventional family and even heterosexuality itself.

For some women, therefore, engaging with feminist analysis led to a denigration of activities particularly associated with women's conventional caring roles, such as nursing. For other women, the feminist emphasis on the importance of individual women's opportunities and freedoms conflicted with the importance they placed on their own caring roles and activities in support of their home and family. Under Margaret Thatcher's Conservative Governments 1979–90, discourses around the family and personal relationships changed, emphasising responsibility rather than individual freedoms. Pro-family organisations grew in influence, alongside what was described as a 'New Right' emphasis on traditional social structures. Somerville (*op. cit.*) explores the development of what she sees as two women's movements, one linked to ideologies of feminism, Marxism and liberalism and the other linked to Christianity and conservatism. She suggests that how women understand their experience 'depends on different access to and engagement with discourses through which meanings are constructed about the nature of the individual and social relations, of social hierarchies, of sexuality and sexual difference, of personal identity and social responsibility' (*ibid.*: 690). Access to a range of discourses may depend in part on access to educational opportunities.

Nursing's history, as Denny has illustrated in Chapter Four, means that nursing has strong links to Christianity and to a class based conservatism. Although nursing has engaged with feminism, feminism's influence seems to have been largely confined to education, with little impact on practice (Webb 2002). The persistence of stereotypical images of nurses in the media in Britain ensures the endurance of discourses which assign women sexual, decorative, domestic and subordinate roles. Nursing's close associations with women's traditional roles may have made it comparatively difficult for nurses to engage with broader debates about women's role. Hallam (1998) has noted that although the social diversity of women entering nursing increased in the latter half of the 20th century, higher class women seeking higher education and professional roles sought opportunities outside nursing.

Middle class families took advantage of the expansion of higher education in the 1960s to ensure their daughters gained access to the advantages of a university education. As opportunities for women to work increased through changing discourses about women's role, professional families recognised the importance of higher education for their daughters' ability to gain and retain status advantage. Girls with 'A' levels increasingly rejected nursing and favoured other professions, including medicine. Even now women appear to continue to depend overwhelmingly on the education process to secure their position in the labour market, whereas boys have a range of other resources on top of their qualifications. Savage and Egerton (*op. cit.*: 667) found that 'The class privileges of daughters depend overwhelmingly on their scoring well on ability tests and then (presumably) using credentialist methods to sustain their class advantages.'

Class differences in discourses about education as well as about women's role and other skills may have affected nursing through a complex process of women judging women. The initial difficulties of gaining access to male dominated professions such as medicine and the law could have led women choosing such difficult routes to denigrate other women's choices, seeing such choices as failing to value women's progress, women's higher education and the rewards of social position. Nurses may not necessarily share such values. Within nursing, differing levels of qualifications led to different interest groups. Nursing history demonstrates that conflict between different groups of nurses has been common.

Nurse education and higher education

Nursing was relatively slow to seek the advantages of a university education. However some universities launched pre-registration degrees in the 1970s and post-registration health visiting and nurse teacher courses had been offered within colleges and universities from the early decades of the 20th century. The first nursing professorship was established at the University of Edinburgh in 1971. By 1989, fifteen higher education institutions offered extended undergraduate courses leading to a first degree in nursing and a first level nursing qualification; however, at that time, the number of nursing graduates remained insignificant, at only three per cent of nursing qualifiers per annum (Lelean and Clarke 1990). Nursing finally sought entry into higher education through the Project 2000 nurse education reforms, proposed and agreed in the

1980s (UKCC *op. cit.*). The profession argued that student nurses should be students not workers and academic recognition was sought through gaining higher education diploma level status for the profession's entry level qualification.

Part of the ideology which accompanied arguments for educational reform was the view that nursing could be seen as an autonomous profession, taking responsibility for patients through a system of organising nursing care which allowed an individual nurse to take responsibility for patients (primary nursing). The primary nurse would be assisted by associate nurses. Advocates of this new model of the nurse–client relationship saw 'new nursing' as being underpinned by an education which provided opportunities for personal growth as well as knowledge development and skills of reflective practice, of research and of decision making (Salvage 1992). An improved education system, it was thought, would attract better educated recruits and provide autonomous practitioners. The profession's success in gaining Government approval for Project 2000 can be seen as a considerable achievement for nursing and a considerable achievement for the education leaders as opposed to nurses responsible for the management of the service. Kitson (2001) notes, however, that the Conservative Government, in introducing the reforms, was indifferent to the ideology (exemplified by primary nursing) concerning nursing professional autonomy and the changing nature of the relationship with the patient. She suggests that governments are interested in their own reform agendas and that 'professional interests are totally dispensable if they are not part of a government agenda' (*ibid.*: 95). The Conservative Government agenda in the 1980s may have included improving the efficiency and effectiveness of nurse education in order to improve the skills of the workforce, but it did not include developing a newly empowered profession capable of expanding its role and status within health care. Kitson suggests that the Labour Government's modernisation agenda, however, provides nursing with many opportunities to benefit (DoH 2000).

Initial doubts about the success of Project 2000 focussed on the preparation of diplomates for professional practice (DoH 1999a, UKCC 1999). Concerns about academic emphasis and lack of practical skills continued throughout the incorporation of nurse education into higher education during the 1990s. Reviews underlined the importance of practical skills, leading to recommendations to change curricula to reduce the perceived theory–practice gap through integrated curricula and longer placements, with the aim of ensuring continued recognition of the importance of clinical skills (DoH *op. cit.*, UKCC *op. cit.*). As already mentioned, Thompson and Watson (*op. cit.*) have argued that there is a danger of overemphasising the importance of short term educational outputs and weakening the educational foundation which develops nursing's critical abilities.

Nurse education literature worldwide reflects different discourses within nursing concerning the nature of nursing skills and appropriate educational processes. What is often not identified within nursing literature is the positional conflict and protectionism that lies behind these views as well as the ongoing influence of assumptions about nurses' natural activities as performing tasks and providing care.

Discourses amongst nurse educators

Studies of nurse educators' strategies for coping with the change from vocational training to academic education suggest that educators have varied views of knowledge and competence. Philhammar Andersson (1999) studied nurse teachers' perceptions of competence in a University in Sweden. She identified three coping strategies which reflected differing emphases on nursing skills and knowledge. Some teachers highlighted the importance of being a 'real' nurse and sought to maintain competence in the working operations and methods of nursing work. For these educators, nursing 'is primarily a practice profession, requiring manual dexterity, a kind heart and a minimum of scientific knowledge' (*ibid.*: 36) (in class terms, this definition would place nursing amongst the skilled manual workers). A second group of nurse teachers stressed the importance of specialised knowledge in academic subject areas (sociology, philosophy, psychology, biological sciences), thus giving prominence to claims to professional status.

A third group emphasised research, theory development and higher degrees such as PhDs in nursing. This group believed that 'only they can change nursing education from vocational training to an academic education' (*ibid.*: 36). This group could be seen as attempting to create a new definition of essential resources for high status autonomous roles in nurse education and practice. The implication is that some nurses could attain a professional status equivalent to that of doctors and lawyers. Philhammar Andersson (*ibid.*: 36) notes that:

> at one level these nurse educators are welcomed among faculty and students as evidence of the professionalization of nursing and they provide the school with an image of an academic setting. In another way they are met with scepticism and fear.

As we have seen, such scepticism about academic achievement has a long history. It may, however, also be understandable if such professionalisation is seen as creating a new form of closure, denying access to high rewards to diverse groups. The second group of educators, those who emphasised the importance of knowledge not 'owned' by nurses, may also perceive that restrictive views about possible membership of an élite nursing group may in fact inhibit nursing's progress through making communication with other élite groups more difficult. Nurse educators in higher education, for example, can highlight their membership of a broader group, that of higher education lecturers. Similarly, nurse managers may give prominence to their membership of a wider health service management community. These are all discourses and strategies which are themselves shaped by social stratification.

Discourses about education

Discourses about the general purposes of education provide a useful framework for considering nurse education. The liberal view of the purpose of education attaches importance to individual development. In this view education is a means of ensuring a meritocratic division of labour based on open and fair competition. As in functionalism (see Chapter One), such a view sees education as a means whereby individuals can

choose to develop their abilities according to their preferences, leading to an efficient and effective method of social
selection. Critiques of what Brown (2000) terms the liberal
account of positional competition argue that groups with
social status find ways of restricting access to opportunities
such as university education and professional training to ensure
their own social group retains advantage. As Brown (*ibid.*:
635) notes, drawing on the ideas of Weber (1945) and
Murphy (1984):

> in these terms modern examination systems represent an example of
> exclusionary closure in a downward direction when one group secures
> its advantage by closing off the opportunities of another group
> beneath it that it defines as inferior or ineligible.

Parkin (1979) has argued that although social groups such
as the aristocracy have lost much of their exclusionary control,
social closure remains significant, with a shift towards 'indi-
vidualist' rather than 'collectivist' rules. This means that individual credentials rather than group membership are vital to
achieving occupational status.

Exclusionary power on the part of groups, such as professional bodies, however, can still be used in varied ways.
Education funding mechanisms may also, for example, limit
access to opportunities to develop the capacities necessary to
develop professional and individual confidence and competence. Concern that funding nursing and allied health professional education through the Department of Health rather
than through the Higher Education Funding Councils inhibited research development in nursing has led to a task force
which explored the prospects for the development of research
capacity in nursing and the allied professions. There is now a
clear recognition that without research capacity building, the
professional capacity of nursing and other health professions
will remain underdeveloped (HEFCE 2001).

One purpose of education is to provide the necessary skills
for the labour market. The changing nature of the labour
market in developed countries has led to increased demand for
higher education. The growth of the middle class has been
fuelled by increased demand for technical, managerial and
professional skills. Employment demands involve not just an

increased volume and level of technical competence but also broader skills such as problem solving, communication, teamwork and self management skills and an ability to manage personal and organisational change. Access to educational opportunities which support the transferable skills necessary for success in a global economy remains competitive. Some forms of selective education, such as Britain's public schools, are seen as particularly successful in developing these skills. It is not clear, however, whether theory based higher education has successfully developed the skills which will lead to positional power in a global economy.

Hirsch (1977) has distinguished between forms of positional power that derive from gaining more resources which are valued *in* the marketplace, and positional power gained through changing the rules *of* the marketplace, particularly by gaining monopolistic power over markets. Brown (*op. cit.*: 637) refers to this distinction as a distinction between 'competition "ranking" (resources in the marketplace) and competition "rigging" (influences over markets)'. He identifies three relevant rules for inclusion and exclusion: membership, meritocratic and market. 'Membership' rules include forms of exclusion and inclusion based on ascribed attributes such as gender, ethnicity, social class; 'meritocratic' rules 'are based on the ideology of individual achievement in an "open" and "equal" contest' (*ibid.*: 639), and 'market' rules are based on supply and demand. The market rules are seen as working in a global context, thus leading to a governmental emphasis on the importance of a highly skilled and educated workforce to ensure that those with the highest credentials can gain access to key positions in an international arena. Brown suggests that the increased use of market rules relating to credentialism and 'the competition for a livelihood has taken the character of a civil war within the middle classes as they strive for the same credentials from élite institutions' (*ibid.*: 648).

The global competitiveness of Britain depends, in part, on the skills of the workforce. This has led to an increasing emphasis on competency based education. Chapman (1999: 130) has argued that 'Most developed countries are experiencing a restructuring of their education curricula on a national standardized basis.' This restructuring has been based on economic rationalism, seen by Chapman as responsible for the introduction of competency based standards. The introduction of National Care Standards is an obvious example in Britain. Competency based education has been described as a means of social closure, 'a strategy of governance, a means of producing consent without the need for oppression and force in the reproduction of the social order' (Edwards and Usher 1994: 2).

It is helpful to consider the competency debate in the context of broader theories about work. Competency based education is viewed with particular scepticism by public service workers who have a long tradition of trust based relations with employers. Welfare professionals, in particular, have been described as politically and socially distinctive in terms of their views about capitalist societies. Webb (1999: 749) suggests, following Bagguley (1995) and Heath and Savage (1995) that 'Self-selection into occupations according to pre-existing political beliefs and values results in a public-sector middle class with a critical attitude to corporate capitalism and a moral commitment to a fairer society.' Lash and Urry (1994) have argued that the work of these professionals is being controlled by processes of economic rationalisation which control the costs of public services. These processes are intensification (methods to increase productivity); commodification (applying the logic of the market to services); concentration (centralisation and central government control); and domestication (relocating work from the public to the private sphere). The nature of professional work is changing, leading to differences between members of what has been termed the 'service class'. As a result, Webb (*op. cit.*: 763) argues this group 'appears fragmented between professional management strategists (mainly men)…and devalued welfare professionals (where women are over-represented) espousing "caring values" '. Ezzy (1997: 440) observes that the subjective experience of professional work is changing and that the meaning of work is developed through an interpretative process which draws on 'pre-existing cultural discourses that frame the experience of work. The narrative also locates working with reference to a broader life plan and purpose that integrally involves the fulfilment of commitments to other people and to society.' It is interesting to consider nursing's move to higher education in the light of these arguments. It is unclear whether nurse education prepares nurses for the complexity of professional work in public services. Davies *et al.* (2000) found no evidence that Project 2000 changed recruitment patterns by attracting more academically qualified recruits into nursing.

Nurse education discourses: nurse education and social trends

As already identified, nurse education literature reflects different discourses about education and different views about the importance of competency based or liberal education.

Competency based education

Nurse education has always attached importance to preparing a competent practitioner, perhaps through an understanding of the need to maintain market position through ensuring nursing recruits are appropriately skilled. Hence nurse education has embraced competency based education. Chapman (1999: 131) is sceptical about the appeal of competency based approaches to education, seeing them as potentially restrictive in highlighting the importance of 'hands-on' nursing care. She suggests:

> the cogent appeal of the competency based approach may seduce nurse educators into advancing the scientific or technical aspects of nursing knowledge at the expense of the artistic or humanistic aspects.

Chapman discusses the inherently conservative nature of competency based education, perhaps driven by its assessment methods, which may mean 'it is easier to value competencies that can be produced, reproduced, assessed and measured according to plan' (*ibid.*: 132). Competency based education may also suppress aspirations to achievement. Chapman sees competency based education as a potential enemy of excellence and progress. Grundy (2001: 262), on the other hand, places the development of the competency based approach to professional education more firmly in the context of criticisms of too much 'academic self interest and indulgence in what will be taught and not enough attention to workplace competence'. As such, a lack of attention to workplace competency derives from an élitist willingness to allow 'the best to be the enemy of the good' (Robertson *op. cit.*: 12). Grundy (*op. cit.*) is optimistic that the limitations of a reductionist, behaviourist approach to outcome competencies (Milligan 1998) can be overcome through higher education institutions defining the process of achieving competency in such a way that education ensures students are confident in both knowledge and skills. The competency based approach can help widen access to nursing through links to National Vocational Qualifications but Grundy also sees it as compatible with role and practice developments in nursing.

Liberal views of educational development

Gillis *et al.* (1998), on the other hand, explore the development of competencies of liberal education in Canadian nurses studying for a nursing baccalaureate, and conclude that 'fundamental in educational reform is the development of baccalaureate programmes for post-RN learners that focus as much on the development of the individual as a person as on the development of the professional nurse' (*ibid.*: 410). This emphasis on a liberal view of the importance of education in individual development reflects a belief that restricted views of skills competency will not broaden and widen opportunities for nurses individually or collectively.

Nursing and policy change

The importance of these debates for nursing at the beginning of the 21st century lies in the opportunities presented by the Labour Government's modernisation agenda (DoH 2000). *The NHS Plan* calls for modernised education and training with a core curriculum for all health professionals to enable practitioners, particularly nurses, to develop new skills and take on new roles. The modernisation agenda includes a new approach to workforce planning to ensure health care services are integrated with other services, particularly social services, in a way which is sensitive to clients' needs and expectations, including expectations of being involved in decisions about their care. The Department of Health recognises difficulties in changing the practices of established staff groups, supported by established career and status hierarchies. Such groups are likely to adopt closure and exclusionary tactics in order to preserve the status quo. The consultation document on the review of workforce planning, *A Health Service of All the Talents: Developing the NHS Workforce* (DoH 2001f), notes that innovative approaches to care have rarely received national support because 'there was often perceived resistance to skill-mix changes, both among clinical middle managers who were uneasy about staff who followed varied career paths and among staff concerned about "dumping" of tasks' (*ibid.*: 21).

The Department of Health proposes to support change and development through a framework for lifelong learning for the NHS based on a clear Government vision. This vision is explained in *Working Together — Learning Together: A Framework for Lifelong Learning for the NHS* (DoH 2001c). The vision includes identifying a set of core values and skills which should be central to lifelong learning in the NHS and health care more generally; an entitlement to work in an environment which equips staff with the skills to perform their current jobs to the best of their ability; and open and flexible access to education, training and development. The document recommends that wherever possible learning should be shared by different staff groups and professions; and that planning and evaluation of lifelong learning should be central to organisational development and service improvement, thus ensuring that learning is valued, recognised, recorded and accredited (*ibid.*: 6).

This is a substantial challenge to features of the existing education system which involves restrictions on access to professional programmes, place of delivery and modes of accreditation, particularly for high status professions. There is also a clear demarcation of roles for doctors, nurses and allied health professions and limited, although growing, movement across professional boundaries and across health and social care. Central to the Department of Health's vision is reform of the regulatory bodies; pay modernisation; modernising jobs; and the concept of the skills escalator, according to which individuals (and professional roles) can move up the escalator to achieve their potential. As jobs are reviewed, tasks can be moved up and down the unidisciplinary ladders to ensure that tasks are located at the lowest level of skill/training at which the tasks are competently performed. This opens up possibilities for non-professional support workers to take on more skills and broaden their role. Pay modernisation, a key part of the process of reform, involves an evaluation of jobs in terms of key characteristics such as communication and relationship skills, knowledge, training and experience; analytical and judgment skills; planning and organisational skills; physical skills; responsibilities for client care, for policy and service development, financial and physical resources, human resources, information resources, and research and development; freedom to act; physical, mental, and emotional effort; and working conditions (Waters 2002). The modernisation process can be seen as an attempt not just to change working practices in the NHS, but to break down class barriers which have inhibited expansion in the United Kingdom's educational system.

As ever, what is particularly significant for nursing is the demarcation between nurses and doctors. It is often helpful to consider the dominant group, the doctor's view. In a web based *BMJ* discussion concerning how doctors and nurses might work together more effectively, Richard Smith (2002) alludes to nurses' and doctors' relative positions in the educational hierarchy:

> Doctors and nurses are divided by gender, background, philosophy, training, regulation, money, status, power, and — dare I say it? — intelligence (doctors are usually top of the class, nurses in the middle).

In subsequent discussion Smith regretted his reference to intelligence, but, nevertheless, discussions concerning changing role boundaries identify the restrictive nature of traditional professional recruitment and professional territorialism. Roskell (2002), for example, also in a web based *BMJ* discussion, writes:

> It could be argued that abolishing the distinction between doctors and nurses would promote mutual understanding and enhance teamwork.

This is unlikely. More probably it would see the end of Medicine as a high quality subject, demanding considerable knowledge, personal qualities, and (politically incorrect, but vital) intelligence.

Roskell (*ibid.*) suggests that the questions underlying the debate are:

1 Do we want doctors to be clever people or not? Personally I want mine to be very clever...
2 Should nurses be able to take on doctors' work? Of course, with training and appropriate supervision, if they want to. But unless they have the same level of training as a doctor, they should remain distinct, not a substitute. Arguably 'doctors' work' that does not require specialist training should not be done by a doctor in the first place.

However sceptical Roskell may be about nurses' abilities, he has thus identified the principles of the skills escalator, whereby individuals can move on according to their abilities and work can be delegated down to less qualified staff.

Given a society in which higher education is part of a process necessary for taking on the majority of roles to which society accords high status, the role of the nurse will only be highly valued if it is a role which requires appropriate educational development. Individual nurses will achieve high status through their educational development. Inevitably, for nursing as a profession and for individual nurses, to move up the skills escalator (and up the social class hierarchy), qualification and experience are increasingly necessary; but at the same time, tasks (such as fetching bedpans) will be passed down the escalator to non-professional staff (from a Marxist standpoint, this can be seen as a proletarianisation of professional work). If nurses are to take on more autonomous decision making roles they will need to ensure that their educational skills of critical reasoning, creative and independent judgment are nurtured within appropriate environments of challenge and support. These skills will be enacted in a changing and perhaps contested environment of changing skill mix and moving role boundaries. Part III of this volume provides some examples of innovative nursing practice which aims to reduce inequalities in health and health care.

Part III

Addressing inequalities through nursing practice

6 Class inequalities in mental health nursing

Paul Godin

Introduction

As capitalism displaced feudalism it brought about major social and economic changes. Though social inequalities were no longer held to be natural, unequal distribution of material and symbolic rewards did not disappear in the modern age of Enlightenment; in some respects it intensified. The capitalist free market, in this rapidly industrialising and urbanising age, exposed the poor to greater insecurity, privation and premature death, which Engels proposed was nothing less than 'social murder' by 'the property-holding classes interested in maintaining and prolonging this disorder' (1995 [1844]: 134). Nineteenth century public health reformers drew attention to the strong association between low social class and physical illness. Despite subsequent improvements in living standards and the 20th century development of the National Health Insurance Scheme and the National Health Service (NHS), which reduced financial barriers to health care, research into social class and health has continued to find this association. Since the seminal work of Hollingshead and Redlich (1958) *Social Class and Mental Illness*, in the USA, research has similarly shown low social class to be associated with a higher rate of mental illness. However, the association between low social class and the diagnosis of mental illness was widely acknowledged in Britain before this, as it was mainly the poor who had been interned within the public asylum system of the 19th century.

In Britain, capitalism gave rise to an extensive and ever expanding state control of madness, from which a range of occupations, such as mental health nursing, emerged. The asylum system grew unremittingly in size for one and a half centuries, reaching a high point of 148,000 psychiatric beds in 1954 (Scull 1977). Though the asylum system has now been largely dismantled and only 28,000 psychiatric beds remain in England, there are currently 630,000 people under the care of mental health care professionals (DoH 2001d). In this chapter I consider how the 57,000 registered mental health nurses in Britain might understand and address capitalist class inequalities within their practice. Towards this end I consider another salient feature of the capitalist era, namely 'citizenship'. Though class inequalities and other social divisions of gender, age and ethnicity pervade capitalist society, citizenship has given rise to the democratising idea that human beings, by virtue of their humanity, are born equal. As Marshall (1950) pointed out, it was this idea of natural equality that enabled the progressive development of civil, political and then social rights in the course of capitalism's history. He argued that the development of social rights in the 20th century imposed modifications upon the inequalities that social class generated. The post-Second World War welfare state represented a victory for social citizenship in its fight against social class. I contend that, though capitalist class society has generated inequalities in mental health and the delivery of health care, the development of citizenship, though never having been fully afforded to mental health service users, has positively shaped the regimes of care to which they have been subject. I suggest further that at the present time, as mental health legislation is being reformed, it is essential that mental health nurses value and employ notions of citizenship to inform their practice. Towards this conclusion about how mental health nurses may positively address social class inequalities within mental health care, I first consider the history of how capitalist class society has influenced the understanding, incidence and management of mental illness, with reference to the developing concept of citizenship.

The asylum

In the early 18th century there were fewer than 10,000 people confined as mad in England, but by 1900 this figure had risen to 100,000 (Porter 1992: 120). It was in the 19th century that the majority of the nation's asylums were built. Like the parallel workhouse system, the public asylum system largely accommodated paupers, who were unable to survive the harsh climate of free market capitalist society. Though the asylum system was criticised for its poor rate of cure and the baneful effects it had upon its inmates, these institutions had been modelled upon the more successful practices of 'moral treatment'. Moral treatment, quite literally, attempted to moralise the insane back into sanity through humane, benign disciplinary regimes of care that encouraged self control. Methods of mechanical, physical restraint were replaced with religious and moral teaching and the movement of a moral conscience within patients towards their self restraint. Moral treatment, which simultaneously arose in England, France, Italy and the USA, was highly indicative of the late 18th century era of Enlightenment, in which capitalism was rapidly transforming production and society. This transformation was predicated upon ideas of civil citizenship that allowed freedom to own property, produce goods and services, set contracts and freely participate in open markets. This notion of civil citizenship was founded upon the idea of natural human equality, which gave credibility to the assertion of moral treatment that, though the mad may be irrational, they were still human. Accordingly moral treatment challenged traditional ideas of the mad being bestial, asserting instead a new sensitivity towards the insane that rather understood them as misguided, deluded and childlike. They were thus capable of being disciplined and instructed towards reason, civility and a productive existence. Foucault (1971) suggested this taming of the mad was even more repressive than preceding treatment regimes that had only sought to control their bodies. Moral treatment, he argued, marked the beginning of mental medicine in the modern era, in which bourgeois reason finally silenced the mad in its control of their bodies and minds. Yet moral treatment favourably improved conditions of treatment and prospects for rehabilitation for its patients. In England, William Tuke pioneered moral treatment at the York Retreat and, as Digby (1985) points out, many patients recovered their senses and were successfully discharged to lead lives as productive citizens. In short, the ideas of civil freedom of the age of Enlightenment and capitalist development inspired moral treatment to bring about a progressive approach in the treatment of the mad.

It was not only ideological changes associated with the rise of capitalism that assisted the development of moral treatment; economic forces within capitalism may also be understood to have promoted the practices of moral treatment. Warner (1985) suggests that the intensive rehabilitative efforts of moral treatment in the USA during the early 19th century were economically motivated as there was then a national labour shortage. However, in England, social class interests and the processes of capitalist class society prevented the replication of moral treatment within the public asylums. Most of the inmates of the public asylums were pauper lunatics who were afforded little respect. It was commonly believed in the Victorian era that both poverty and mental illness were caused by degeneracy that was brought about by amoral conduct, which weakened the constitution. These social Darwinian ideas were clearly expressed by eminent psychiatrists of this time, such as Henry Maudsley, who promoted the belief that mental illness could be passed on from one generation to the next, worsened by degenerative behaviour. Therefore, not only were the mad seen as responsible for their own downfall but they were seen also as a threat to human evolutionary development. Though the asylum system had been founded with great charitable concern to adequately care for the mad, antagonistic Victorian attitudes towards the poor had a countervailing influence. The public asylums were funded out of local taxation. It was therefore hardly surprising that as voting rights were restricted to property owning tax payers, they voted for economies in spending within the asylums. The asylums became overcrowded, understaffed, custodial and devoid of therapeutic optimism.

The poorest members of society lost more than they gained from the new civil freedoms of the enlightened age of capitalism. Dispossessed of the land the urban poor, the proletariat, were forced to sell their labour for less than its true value in order to acquire the basic means of subsistence. Under such conditions relatives of mentally disabled people could not afford to care for them and these members of the lumpenproletariat were forced to seek refuge in the public asylums.

Thus Scull (1979) argues that the asylums became a dumping ground for those who could not survive in the uncompromising free market system of capitalist society. However, one occupational group gained from the growth of the asylum system, achieving professional status and power, dominating patients and nurses. Scull asserts that in defining pathology within mental deviants, incarcerating and managing them within asylums, psychiatrists played a vital role in the state control of that which threatened capitalism. As psychiatrists gained greater control of the asylum system they expanded their empires by increasing the inmate population. Shorter (1997), however, argues that this was rather a response to a rising incidence of mental illnesses, such as schizophrenia, alcohol related disease and tertiary syphilis, which were all generated by the conditions of 19th century capitalist society.

The mental hospital

By the end of the 19th century a large scale, state funded mental health service, in the form of the public asylum system, had developed to control a population of pauper lunatics, confined in impoverished conditions. The 1890 Lunacy Act displayed little concern for the welfare of inmates. It mainly functioned to ensure that nobody's civil rights were violated by wrongful certification and committal to an asylum. Through the 1930 Mental Treatment Act decisions about compulsory detention and treatment shifted decisively towards medicine. Rogers and Pilgrim (1996) contend that this medicalisation of madness effectively weakened civil rights as it made for detention and treatment without trial. However, in renaming lunatics as mental patients and asylums as mental hospitals, the Act arguably improved the status and conditions of those on the receiving end of care. Busfield (1986) proposes that this greater medicalisation of madness made community care conceivable, for if madness was a form of illness, not too dissimilar to physical illness, mental patients, like general hospital patients, could be successfully treated, discharged and even treated in the community. The Act marked the beginning of the greater integration of mental health care into mainstream health care. The renamed institutions became municipal hospitals and were later absorbed into the NHS, as it was born in 1948. Though the compulsory detention of inmates still applied to 90 per cent of inpatients in the 1930s, voluntary status gradually became more common. This trend was promoted further as mental hospitals began unlocking their doors in the 1940s, allowing patients greater parole. The 1959 Mental Health Act consolidated this trend, affording voluntary status to over 90 per cent of mental hospital inpatients. The stigma of being a mental hospital patient was consequently not quite as severe as it had once been. By the 1960s mental hospital patients had a legal, social and moral status far closer to that of patients in a general hospital and of people in wider society.

However, the Victorian ideology of social Darwinism, that had been used to support practices of class discrimination in the treatment of mental patients, continued into the 20th century and in some respects even worsened. The science of eugenics found expression in psychiatry. In the asylums of Nazi Germany methods of euthanasia were developed and then transferred to extermination camps. By 1930, some 24 American states had laws on their statute books allowing for the forced sterilisation of the mental disordered (Kevles 1985). Though eugenics was never formally applied in English mental hospitals, the contempt for those who were thought to threaten human development, promoted by the ideology of social Darwinism, was apparent in the poor treatment of asylum inmates. Lomax (1921), a doctor in Prestwich Asylum during the First World War, poignantly describes the poverty of inmates' existence. They were poorly clothed, inadequately cared for and received insufficient food. This, Lomax argued, led to the high death rate within the nation's asylums, which rose to one in three in a one year period ending in 1919 (Scull 1996) and continued at around ten per cent per year throughout the 1920s and 1930s (Ramon 1985). As many patients were dying in the asylums as were being discharged. However, by the 1950s Government policy improved food and other conditions within mental hospitals, though they were then more overcrowded than ever before. A new pattern of care was then becoming evident as short stay care became far more common. Psychiatry was by now far more committed to the cure of mental illness and less concerned with the mere containment of madness. Jones (1972) talks of there being a threefold revolution in mental health services in the post-Second World War period. Though psychiatrists emphasised the importance of the 'drug revolution' in bringing about the new pattern of care, Jones stresses the greater importance of an administrative revolution, involving the unlocking of mental hospitals and the transformation of how they were run, and a legal revolution, which gave most patients voluntary status.

This revolutionary transition of archaic asylums into hospitals may be identified with a range of factors, not least that psychiatrists were concerned that psychiatry should be acknowledged as a credible and respectable branch of medicine. To this end they actively sought the greater medicalisation and integration of mental health services. I want to draw attention to how the development of capitalist class society and citizenship may be understood to be associated with this mid 20th century revolution in mental health care. As we saw in Chapter One, it can be argued that as capitalist society became more complex in the 20th century, so too did its class structure. Wealth and political control were no longer so decisively held by the bourgeoisie. As Marshall (*op. cit.*) points out, the 19th century witnessed the development of political citizenship, as ever more people gained the right to vote and stand for political office. In the early part of the 20th century trade unionism developed as an influential form of political citizenship that asserted collective demands for basic social rights. In a history of the Confederation of Health Service Employees (CoHSE), traditionally the main trade union for nurses within mental hospitals, Carpenter (1985) argues that it was trade union pressure that brought about improvements in food rations and other conditions for staff and patients within mental hospitals, having to oppose medical superintendents and professional associations, such as the RCN, in the process. Carpenter also contends that CoHSE helped contribute to the birth of the NHS. Trade unionism certainly forced government into securing social rights. The World Wars also undoubtedly pressured government into assuming more responsibilities for the provision of welfare. By the end of the Second World War the welfare state guaranteed British citizens the social right to a universal basic level of welfare. However, as O'Connor (1973) argued, this development of social rights, through the welfare state, also functioned to the advantage of capitalism as it both legitimated capitalism and assisted greater capital accumulation. A healthier, better educated and less impoverished workforce was also more efficient and profitable. Nonetheless the development of welfare capitalism consolidated social citizenship, for though there was still inequality of income and resources the universal right to employment, a basic standard of housing, income, education and health care had been established. In such a world mental hospitals had to lose their associations with previous practices of merely confining pauper lunatics, for social citizenship raised the worth of all human beings, including mental patients. It was no longer acceptable to strip mental patients of their civil selves and institutionalise them in asylums in the fashion that Goffman (1961) so poignantly describes. They were now, like everybody else, social citizens and thus had a right to something better. The political sentiments of the post-Second World War era were reflected in psychiatry, which revised the aspirations of moral treatment towards the rehabilitation of mental patients into open employment and society. Warner (*op. cit.*) argues that this development was economically driven, for there was a post-war labour shortage in Britain. This, he argues, greatly stimulated the rehabilitative efforts of what became known as 'social psychiatry'. As work was a duty of social citizenship, employment helped mental patients towards their social integration. Also, treatment was no longer restricted to those whose poverty and disability forced them into mental hospitals. Psychiatry, now under the NHS, democratically treated anybody identified as having a mental health problem. This wider scope of mental health care services helped erode some of the stigma associated with mental illness.

Community care

Although the asylums had been renamed and reformed they still stood as an embarrassing reminder of the Victorian age.

Announcing Government plans for their demise at MIND's annual conference Enoch Powell, then Minister for Health, referred to them as a 'running sore on the face of civilised society' (MIND 1961). In their place were to be psychiatric units in general hospitals and community care. However, progress towards achieving this ideal was slow. It was not until 1987 that any of the nation's mental hospitals were actually closed and community care remained an under-funded, ill defined and arbitrary practice for decades. Drawing upon O'Connor's thesis, Scull (1977) argues that the move towards community care (a move that he proposes might be better named 'community neglect'), was driven by economic factors. With the post-war welfare infrastructure in place within the community it was feasible to close the old mental hospitals, which were an intolerable financial burden to the capitalist state, particularly when in financial crises. Scull has been accused of being too economistic in his analysis (Sedgwick 1982, Prior 1991). In particular what stands against Scull's theory is the fact that the number of mental health care professionals and spending on mental health care have both increased, despite the closure of mental hospitals.

In most industrialised countries where welfare capitalism developed, sooner or later, so too was there a move towards community care. I suggest that to a greater or lesser extent community care policy and practices have often been motivated by a concern to promote the social worth and citizenship of service users in the process of reshaping the nature of mental health care. The actions of the Marxist inspired Psichiatria Democratica movement in Italy in the 1960s and 1970s provide a good example of this. Basaglia, one of the movement's main exponents, argued that capitalist class society had given rise to a psychiatric system, obscured in an aura of scientific objectivity, which functioned to isolate and contain social problems and class conflicts. Psichiatria Democratica aimed to recast mental health care by eradicating its lynchpin — the asylum — and establish a radical alternative in the community that would not be based upon coercive welfare. Basaglia argued that 'patients had to be given back their rights as citizens' (1981: 187) as a first step towards their rehabilitation. New, democratically run centres for mental health were set up where, Basaglia claimed, 'patients and townsfolk could discover their common interests and oppression' (*ibid.*: 191). In the USA the Kennedy administration attempted to improve mental health care services through a radical community care policy in the 1960s, based upon replacing mental hospitals with community mental health centres (CMHC), which were to offer more preventive and comprehensive mental health care. The CMHC model began to be emulated in Britain during the 1980s. Perhaps the best example of community mental health care policy and practice, demonstrating a concern to promote the social worth and citizenship of service users, was evident in the application of the treatment ideology of 'normalisation' (Wolfensberger 1972), which was applied in the resettlement, to the community, of mental patients from hospitals under closure in the late 1980s and 1990s. The doctrine of normalisation asserted that disabled people had hitherto been marginalised and disempowered, and that it was this disempowerment that services needed to attend to, more than individual pathology. As its slogans stated, it was about 'changing services not people'; professionals being 'on tap not on top'; and 'giving disabled people a more-than-equal chance of participating in civil and economic life'. Normalisation stood in stark opposition to ideas and class discriminatory practices supported by social Darwinism. However, some professionals vigorously opposed normalisation, protesting that it irresponsibly ignored mental patients' psychiatric needs (Clifford 1986). Not only did it threaten professional domination over mental patients, but it also riled many who objected to mental patients being elevated to this new status of normality. Since the era of moral treatment, the full citizenship of mental patients had been contingent upon their recovery. The doctrine of normalisation asserted that irrespective of being mentally ill they were full citizens, entitled to the normal and socially valued life in the community that other people enjoyed. This for some was too much. As Barham puts it: 'Those who scorn normalization are those who want to unmask the mental patient behind the facade of the ordinary person and retrieve him for mental patient-hood' (1992: 150).

As the number of people receiving mental health care increased so too did the number and diversity of mental health professionals. This development of mental health care under the conditions of welfare capitalism, that emphasised social citizenship, enabled mental health care services to move away from the mere containment and control of mental deviants, who were largely from the poorest section of society. However, it would be wrong to conclude that this development entirely militated against social class inequalities in mental health care. As mental health care became more diverse and comprehensive, class inequalities in treatment became ever more evident. Put simply, softer and more desirable treatments, such as psychotherapy, were more often given to less severely mentally ill people, who were usually from the middle classes, whilst harsher and less desirable treatments, such as major tranquillisers, often coercively administered, were more frequently visited upon the severely mentally ill people, who were more inclined to be of low social class. It has been argued that the stress of poverty, lack of opportunity and social disorganisation experienced by people of low social classes renders them more inclined to suffer psychosis (Faris and Dunham 1967). It has also been suggested that middle class people are more inclined to endure neurotic rather than psychotic illnesses because their upbringing promotes inhibitions, whereas a lower class, less secure and stable upbringing renders people more inclined to a loss and fragmentation of their sense of self, which may develop into psychotic illness (Langer and Michael 1963). Yet middle class mental health professionals may more readily recognise psychoses in working class patients than they do in middle class patients whom they can more easily identify with.

Not only did a class division arise in diagnosis and treatment, based largely upon a psychotic versus neurotic distinction, but also a class ordered division of labour arose within mental health care services. The treatment of psychosis, other than its diagnosis and the prescription of drugs, was generally regarded as menial and dishonourable work as it often involved dirty, coercive tasks. This was largely the province of the psychiatric nurses in hospital. As the number of mental health care workers increased they all clamoured for professional status by concentrating on the cleaner, smarter work of psychotherapy with neurotic short term patients, avoiding work with psychotic long term patients. Sladden (1979), for example, in a study of community psychiatric nurses' (CPNs) practice in Edinburgh, found that, although half of their patients were seen for injections, this took place in depot clinics where patients were quickly dealt with in sessions averaging three minutes, by whichever CPN had the chore of running the clinic on that day. However, CPNs' home visits were much longer in duration and were largely reserved for less severely ill clients. With varying levels of class advantages, doctors, social workers, psychologists, nurses and occupational therapists contested the issue of who was best suited to do the talking therapy and who should care for chronic patients. Class prejudices frequently broke loose in interdisciplinary bickering, highlighting the fact that this was a class conflict between occupational groups competing for professional power. Rae (2000), reviewing the history of community psychiatric nursing, recalls how a consultant psychiatrist once remarked that training CPNs to be counsellors was as ridiculous as teaching lorry drivers to be airline pilots. By the late 1980s such professional class conflict had at least contributed to an embarrassing criticism that mental health care services had to face, namely that the 'inverse care law' (Hart 1971), whereby those in most need of health care receive the least care, seemed to apply in the case of non-coercive mental health care. As a new framework for the delivery of community mental health care took shape so too did the focus of mental health services shift towards a prioritisation of long term patients. This was not simply the result of a sudden enlightenment of mental health care professionals, though many are now clearly converted to the equity and wisdom of such an approach; rather it can be associated with changes in Government mental health policy and broader social changes in the nature of capitalist class society.

New community care

The new framework for the delivery of community mental health of the 1990s was largely based on two systems of case management. First, under 'care management', social services assumed responsibility for the financing of community care.

Secondly, the Care Programme Approach (CPA) developed as a health service led system for managing the health and social needs of all people under the care of specialist mental health care services. Strong emphasis was placed upon prioritising the needs of people with 'severe and enduring mental illness'. Also, following a number of high profile cases of homicides and suicides involving mental patients, mental health professionals were clearly instructed to carry out systematic risk assessments on all their patients and to construct risk management strategies of care. Working with long term patients was suddenly seen as important and professionals were less inclined to dissociate themselves from such work. Though this redressed the inequality of least resources going to those most in need, the services that were now being targeted on long term patients were increasingly to do with their surveillance and control, as need became redefined as risk.

New community care must be understood in the context of how capitalist society had changed in the latter part of the 20th century. In the immediate post-Second World War period the state had become extensively involved in the national economy and welfare provision in what became known as the 'Keynesian welfare state'. By the 1970s, in the face of economic crises, this model of government was no longer held to work. The Thatcher/Major Conservative administrations set about a radical reconstruction of the economy and welfare. Keynesian economics was abandoned for a return to monetarism, and the frontiers of the welfare state were rolled back through policies of privatisation and a less redistributive system of taxation. As the frontiers of the welfare state receded so too did social rights, exacerbating inequalities of wealth that were growing substantially under neoliberal government. A new form of citizenship took shape based on libertarian ideas of personal choice and economic freedom. The Major government refused to adopt the European Social Chapter, that would have established social rights, such as a minimum wage, and instead asserted a 'Citizens' Charter', suggesting that citizenship was not about social solidarity and welfare but was rather about the free exercise of personal choice as a consumer.

Housing policy provides a clear example of how a neoliberal government's rolling back of the welfare state was promoted as a means of advancing citizenship, though it increased inequalities of wealth and had a very negative effect on the incidence of mental illness. A study by Nettleton and Burrows (1998) found that people with mortgage arrears had substantial mental health problems. The privatisation of social housing was attractively presented as the 'right to buy', at below market prices, for local authority property tenants. Saunders (1990b) argued that this would create a more secure future for them and means of access to a better quality of life. However, the poorest tenants, who could not afford to buy, could not benefit from the sell-off. Furthermore, the reduction of social housing, along with greater unemployment and poverty, considerably increased homelessness. Yet, despite the fact that discharged patients of closing mental hospitals were largely reprovided for in community residential care schemes, in the context of neoliberal politics, homelessness was blamed on them and on the community care policy that had allowed them out of the asylums. Though a high incidence of mental illness has been found amongst homeless people this was rather the result of homelessness itself. The threat of homelessness, faced by many in the mid 1990s, for whom home ownership was becoming unsustainable, made for their poorer mental health.

A new class order with new ideas about the nature of citizenship took form in a neoliberalist era. Traditional industries, often with communities built around them, which had sustained working class identity, rapidly declined. In what has been characterised as the shift from Fordist to post-Fordist capitalism, the focus changed from production to consumption. Accordingly, people have less of a sense of traditional work based class identity as they derive a greater sense of identity from what they consume. Therefore, although the wealth gap between rich and poor greatly increased in the neoliberal era, class society has arguably disappeared. In its place has arisen a more individualised society based on privatised consumption and individual responsibility. Welfare entitlements, such as housing, pensions and education, have been increasingly eroded. Provision of welfare has progressively passed from the state to individuals, who are now expected to be actively self governing, entrepreneurial and prudent in securing their own health and welfare. However, although traditional class structures, based on our relationship to production, may have disappeared, society has become noticeably more socially divided in terms of wealth and security. As Hutton (1995) argued, neoliberal society enabled the 30 per cent of society at the top to get richer, the 30 per cent at the bottom to become worse off and the 40 per cent in the middle to become 'newly insecure', facing greater risk of losing their home or job and more exposed to privation as the welfare state was being rolled back. Thus, neoliberalism could be understood as having created more losers than winners; not only are those at the bottom comparatively worse off financially, the erosion of the welfare state made for the erosion of their social citizenship. Furthermore, the neoliberalist emphasis upon individual choice and responsibility made for a more individualistic and unfriendly society in which positive attitudes towards the less well off were in short supply. Mental patients, largely in the community, predominantly on low income, now had to endure the backlash against community care, which vilified them as a dangerous risk to society. This has exposed them to considerable hostility. In a MIND questionnaire survey of service users, that yielded 778 respondents, 14 per cent stated that they had been physically attacked, 25 per cent felt at risk of attack in their own home, and 26 per cent said they had been forced to move home because of harassment (Read and Baker 1996). In a recent interview survey in Northern Ireland (McKenna 2000) mental health service users described their experience of victimisation. At home they reported experiences of neighbours daubing graffiti on the walls of their homes, bricks being thrown at their doors and through their windows, and visits from paramilitaries demanding that they move. They reported being spat at, verbally abused in public places and being robbed after cashing their benefit giro cheques.

In many respects in contemporary society we are exposed to innumerable hazards. As Beck (1992) asserts, we live in a 'risk society'. Though science and industrialisation have controlled many aspects of our world they have also exposed us to a wider range of incalculable new dangers. Furthermore, we are now more exposed to the changing fortunes of capitalism against which the Keynesian welfare state government once provided some security. In a world of hazards, Beck argues, we are divided less by class than by our exposure to risk. It is ironic that mental health service users, who are already exposed to a great deal of privation and risk, become scapegoated as a source of danger and are thereby exposed to the additional risk of abuse from the public.

A third way

It might have been hoped that with the election of a Labour government in 1997, committed to a revision of mental health care policy, the fortunes of mental health service users might have improved. Yet there has been no reduction in the wealth gap and only minor and uneven restoration of state welfare. Though the New Labour government's mental health policy has involved a rise in spending on mental health care, a large proportion of this money has been identified for forensic inpatient services in the custody of the few rather than the care of the many. The Government's anti-poverty strategy aims not to redistribute wealth but rather to enable people, through a 'hand up' rather than 'handouts', to help them find their own way out of poverty. 'Handouts', such as Disability Living Allowance, that many mental health service users rely on, have been vigorously restricted.

The New Labour government presented its 'third way' as a viable solution to a world changed by globalisation. Old Labour policies of 'tax and spend' were declared to be unsuited to this changed world and neoliberal government had putatively proved itself unwilling properly to manage change. New Labour promised to restore control and to build a decent, fair and more civil society, though this was not to be achieved through socialist methods of wealth redistribution. I suggest that mental health service users are becoming losers in this managed, morally sound New Labour utopia. Not only is there little hope of them being any wealthier but also they stand to lose rights of citizenship.

New Labour's concept of citizenship is quite similar to that of the neoliberals. Though we are to expect good standards from the public services this is not because we have social rights to a universal level of welfare, but rather because we have, as modern consumers, become accustomed to demanding and receiving high quality services in the private sector and should rightly now expect them of public services too. New Labour, however, now intent upon managing change and 'modernising' public services, portrayed the Thatcher/Major administration as having allowed too many freedoms, resulting in the social exclusion of many and a disorderly society. Frank Dobson (then Secretary of State for Health), announcing the New Labour mental health care policy as a 'third way' beyond the failures of the old asylum system and mismanagement of community care, proclaimed that the latter had 'failed' and gone 'too far', as discharged mental patients had been left to 'wander' and become 'a nuisance and danger to themselves and others' (DoH 1998a). To restore order new mental health legislation was proposed to secure the preventive detention of people who have 'dangerous and severe personality disorders' and ensure that patients in the community comply with treatment, through new compulsory treatment orders that could be applied beyond the hospital. One of the aims of the National Service Framework for Mental Health has been to reduce social exclusion amongst mental health service users, through health promotion aimed at reducing stigma and discrimination (DoH 1999b). Yet New Labour has pandered to popular prejudices about mental patients 'wandering' out of control in the community. It is proposed to enact legislation to further curtail the civil freedoms of mental patients, which will surely leave them more rather than less socially excluded.

Conclusion

What, then, may be learnt from the history of mental health care within capitalist class society? What lessons might the mental health nurses of today draw from it? It is certainly apparent that large scale state funded mental health care, with the occupations of psychiatry and mental nursing that it created, arose in the era of capitalism to control the threat madness posed to social and economic order. This history also shows that although mental health professionals are agents of social control they have variously discharged this function. On the one hand they have augmented their patients' suffering and position of social class disadvantage. Class prejudice against mental patients, supported by social Darwinian ideology, was realised in the practices of their privation, starvation, sterilisation and euthanasia in the late 19th and early 20th centuries. Mental health professionals are also guilty of often securing their own social class advantage at the expense of their clients. Yet on the other hand, they have created and adopted ideologies and practices, such as moral treatment, social psychiatry, Psichiatria Democratica and normalisation, to challenge and redress their clients' social disadvantages. All such movements have placed a high premium on the idea that mental health service users are entitled to citizenship. I suggest that mental health nurses of today who are interested in overcoming rather than adding to their clients' social disadvantages, similarly need to promote and apply notions of citizenship within their practices. The lexicon of third way politics that readily refers to citizenship and related concepts, such as 'social inclusion', needs to be challenged, not least by mental health nurses and others who have to deal with its contradictions at an operational level. One might question, for example, whether the social inclusion of mental health service users is less likely under the New Labour government, given its enthusiasm for extending compulsory treatment into the community and to limit disability living allowance payments. We might also ask how exactly stigma and prejudice towards the mentally ill are to be overcome if Labour politicians talk about patients being left to 'wander' in the community as 'a danger and nuisance to themselves and others'.

In a society divided more by risk than traditional social class it is perhaps more important to understand our clients' social disadvantage in term of their greater exposure to risks in a hostile world that affords them few benefits, and has little sympathy for or understanding of them and, in addition, scapegoats them as a source of danger within the risk society. Rather than going along with society's concerns to scapegoat, marginalise and control mental patients, mental health nurses could play a role in countering this situation. Mental health nurses could challenge the shift in mental health policy and practice towards understanding service users' needs in terms of the risks they pose to social order, which has occurred over the past decade. This shift has emphasised mental health nurses' social control function and discouraged concern about the risks patients face from a hostile, unfriendly society and from iatrogenic mental health treatment. I suggest that mental health nurses could pay more attention to these latter risks that their patients face in their construction of risk assessment and risk management plans, which might then redirect their practice away from coercion rather towards care. This could be justified by reference to ideals within nursing about providing 'holistic care' and values declared within government mental health policy such as clients' right to involvement as a partner within their care and treatment, needing to overcome social exclusion. Thus mental health service users could be understood as citizens, with individual preferences and needs that should be taken into account, rather than as mere objects of risk. These needs of clients might then be less readily subordinated to mental health care policy's overwhelming concerns about 'safety' and the over-exaggerated risk of mental patients to society. Mental health nurses might also form a stronger alliance with user groups and together lobby for care rather than coercion and against the custody of the few at the expense of caring for the many. In both practice and political action mental health nurses could fight against the socially divisive effects of capitalism that leave their clients in such disadvantaged circumstances, by reasserting their social rights. History shows us that this can result in some limited and temporary success. It is, perhaps, a battle that continually needs to be fought, against the socially divisive effects of capitalism.

7 Inequalities in the provision of children's health services

Valerie Watson

Introduction

Children's health services have a significant impact on the care delivered to children by health care professionals. Children in Britain are being disadvantaged through factors ranging from basic disagreements as to the definition of a child to the wide discrepancies in the delivery of children's services nationally. This is in spite of governmental support for 'family values' and the recognition that investing in children's health reaps long term benefits for the health of the future adult population. There are many aspects of current policy provision influencing these inequalities. However this chapter discusses only some of the most contentious, including policies relating to poverty, access to health care, and provision of health services for children. Evidence presented here suggests that today as well as in a historical context, inequalities in the provision of children's health and nursing services mirror inequalities in the care of our children within British society in the 21st century.

Inequalities in health

There is significant evidence that, as with adults, a class gradient exists in relation to both mortality and morbidity in children and young people (Acheson 1998). Until recently, one of the most influential political explanations for these phenomena was lifestyle choice amongst the lower social classes, as exemplified by the *The Health of the Nation* strategy, adopted by the Conservative Government led by John Major (DoH 1992). However, advocates for children and young people argued that they have little or no influence over the lifestyle choices available to them and that such choices are made for them predominantly by their parents, guardians or carers. More recently the Labour government's position on the nation's health, explained in the Green Paper *Our Healthier Nation*, encouraged local authorities to set targets for health improvements (DoH 1998b), recognising that the health of an individual is not solely determined by lifestyle choices but also by environmental and social factors including poverty. Initiatives such as 'Healthier Schools' have been embraced by some, but not all schools are setting internal targets for improving the health of their pupils. As yet there is little evidence to suggest that this scheme is having an effect on children in schools, and there are no plans to make the scheme mandatory.

According to the Child Poverty Action Group (CPAG) (2001) 20 per cent of children live in low income households, more than in any other social group, and numbers are rising. Newman and Roberts (2001) identify as those most at risk of the consequences of inequalities in health due to poverty looked after children; children from some ethnic minority groups; children in single parent households or households with low incomes; children who experience abuse; those with learning disabilities; those from travelling communities, and refugees.

Examples of the direct consequences for health for families with children living in poverty are numerous. Childhood accidents are the primary cause of mortality in children aged 5–15 years, with children from the poorest families twice as likely to die as children in the highest social classes (CPAG 2001). The most common cause of death (27 per cent) among boys aged 5–15 years is accidents. Among girls, accidents are the second highest cause of mortality in this age group at 17 per cent (Statistics 2001). More recent research indicates that children from Britain's most deprived areas are three times more likely to be victims of pedestrian accidents. Most children who are killed are pedestrians rather than passengers or cyclists (*ibid.*). Even after allowing for the number of children per neighbourhood the poorer wards had 2.2 casualties per 100,000 children compared with 0.6 per 100,000 in the wealthier wards. Despite having a good overall record on road safety compared with other European countries, Britain continues to have a poor record on child safety. Campaigners for improvements in child safety repeatedly call for a lowering of the speed limit to 20 miles per hour around schools, and bigger and better play areas for children in neighbourhoods where children often play unsupervised in the streets. Accident prevention must remain an important subject alongside other areas of health education in the curriculum for children aged 10–13, for whom the incidence of road traffic accidents remains high, as children in this age group demand increasing independence away from adult supervision.

The findings from studies are consistent. Reading *et al.* (1999) demonstrate that attendances at accident and emergency units by pre-school children were much higher in deprived urban neighbourhoods than in affluent areas. They conclude that improved child care facilities and targeted accident prevention are both essential changes required in local and national social policy. Despite continued emphasis on these inequalities, there is little to suggest that local and national governments' policies are prepared to address the situation seriously. Although lower speed limits are to be found in some towns and cities, the rationale for these is often traffic calming measures and general accident prevention, with the provision of child friendly areas in urban districts a costly and low priority addition to services.

Uptake of health and education services

There is some evidence suggesting that there is a low uptake of services available to help children and families in poverty. One in five children are not receiving free school meals for which they are eligible. In a study carried out by the Thomas Coram Research Unit (Storey and Chamberlain 2001) the quality and choice of free food available, plus the embarrassment involved in obtaining free school meals, were significant factors in their refusal. Sub-standard nutrition in childhood can cause failure to develop and grow normally and an increased susceptibility to infection and disease. During the school day a lack of food will cause problems with concentration and ultimately the child's learning capabilities (Brander 2000). The importance of the school meal is highlighted in a policy document published by the then Department for Education and Employment (Storey and Chamberlain *op. cit.*) stating that for many pupils the meal they eat at school is the main meal of the day. One in ten children do not eat breakfast and one in six do not receive a cooked meal in the evening, with children increasingly relying on 'fast foods' and snacks. One possible consequence is the rise of childhood obesity, with ten per cent of children aged 9–11 clinically obese (Cole *et al.* 2000). Doctors are blaming a high fat diet and a lack of exercise in this age group for an increase in such conditions as Diabetes II, a condition usually associated with overweight adults.

Since 1980 there has been no legal requirement for schools to provide a school meals service except for children entitled to free provision. In the last 20 years the school meals service has declined further. Nutritional standards for school meals were reintroduced in April 2001 in response to concern about their quality. However, as contracts for the provision of school meals were renewed and a corresponding price increase ensued, this subsequently caused a significant reduction in the number of children and their families requesting school meals (Storey and Chamberlain *op. cit.*). Many schools are removing the provision of school meals for their pupils as a cost cutting measure, with areas previously used as dining rooms now being used as classrooms. The quantity and quality of food and drink available to children during the school day are currently of concern to many child health professionals. Dehydration causes a lack of concentration during lessons and poor performance during physical exercise. The successful management of childhood enuresis and encoporesis programmes depends on children having access to fluids throughout the day. As a result of their recent survey the Enuresis Resource and Information Centre (Brander *op. cit.*) discovered that only one school in ten had freely available drinking water for their pupils. A campaign for drinking water to be freely available for all school age children has resulted in free information packs being sent to hundreds of schools. There remains no compulsion for schools to provide anything for children to eat or drink.

Mayall (1994) compares the rights of children at primary school with those of factory workers. Factory workers have certain rights accorded to them by the Health and Safety at Work Act 1992, whereas school aged children have none. The discrepancies in workers' and children's rights include environmental temperature, provision of drinking water and the provision of toilets. Mayall found that even children aged four years were not allowed to access the toilet when they wanted to but could only use the toilets during breaks for fear that they were trying to get out of working. Mayall concurs with Brander's later findings that a poor daily fluid intake plus restricted access to toilets increases the incidence of enuresis, encoporesis and constipation in this age group (Brander *op. cit.*).

On average 15,400 babies are born annually weighing between 1000 and 2000 grams (CPAG *op. cit.*). These low birth weight and pre-term babies are more likely to be born to young, poor mothers who often have difficulties accessing appropriate health services, for example, antenatal appointments and antenatal classes (Baird 1999). Low birth weight and pre-term babies are more at risk of long term health care problems due to their immaturity and weak immune systems. Long term problems include increased risk of infection during the first year, especially respiratory infections exacerbated by the damp environments typically found in poor housing conditions. Due to advances in neonatal medicine more low birth weight babies are surviving. These babies often require access to specialist health care services such as disability services, incurring additional financial and social costs for their families (Bissell 2002). Specialist community neonatal nurses are available in some areas to support families of sick pre-term babies; however there is no national provision. Also, due to the demands of their workload, the specialist nurses often visit these families for a limited period of time. Longer term support depends on community nursing services. In some areas these community nurses are adult trained nurses lacking in the knowledge of the specialist needs of sick children and their carers. The lack of a comprehensive children's community nursing service in England and Wales contributes to the inequality of access to a holistic service for these children and their families (Muir and Sidey 2000).

Key health personnel such as children's nurses, community paediatricians, school nurses and health visitors have important roles to play in determining local health promotion policies. However this chapter demonstrates that these services are considered to be low priority health services, at risk of underfunding. Acheson (1998) and Newman and Roberts (*op. cit.*) identify health care workers such as health visitors as personnel working at the interface with local families and communities who can make a real difference in tackling inequalities in health.

Implications for children's nursing

Children and young people make up 20 per cent of the population (Statistics 2001) and yet resources such as nursing and health services for this age group are sparse compared to other age groups (Whiting 1998). As the majority of children and young people live in families who traditionally have a responsibility of care towards them (a responsibility reinforced by The Children Act 1989), there is an expectation that such health care will predominantly take place within the family.

The Platt Report (Ministry of Health 1959) highlighted the importance of children being nursed by qualified children's nurses and these recommendations have been reinforced ever since, most notably in The Clothier Report (DoH 1994) and The Kennedy Report (Kennedy 2001). However, there remains a dearth of qualified children's nurses. Areas experiencing particular problems in recruiting and retaining qualified children's nurses are those areas deemed to be predominantly adult services such as accident and emergency departments and intensive care units (DoH 1997, Royal College of Paediatrics and Child Health (RCPCH) 1999). Other areas where there are insufficient specialist children's nurses to meet demand are in community settings, where the need for a unique children's community nursing service has been a recent phenomenon (Muir and Sidey *op. cit.*).

Children accessing health services are faced with a service designed for adults. General practitioners, dentists, outpatient departments and referral services such as X-ray and phlebotomy services all have an air of clinical efficiency which is likely to be unfamiliar to children. The services are managed and run by practitioners trained to care for the adult population. As a result of recent guidelines encouraging such areas to be more patient friendly (RCPCH *op. cit.*) some have introduced boxes of toys and allocated space as children's areas, where children can wait with other children.

The Royal College of Paediatrics and Child Health, in conjunction with the Royal College of Nursing and Action for Sick Children, have reviewed the accident and emergency services for children across the country. The working party found that 25–30 per cent of attendees at accident and emergency departments were children. Whilst recognising that there were an increasing number of examples of good practice, these were not found to be universal. The review concludes that there were 'inequalities in health care for the most vulnerable members of society in the most urgent of situations' (RCPCH *op. cit.*: 6). Their recommendations include the audiovisual separation of children from adults; a registered children's nurse on every shift; age appropriate toys available under the supervision of a play specialist; a closer liaison with the primary health care teams; and a greater emphasis on health promotion and accident prevention within departments. Special mention was also made of the lack of facilities and consideration offered to young people, that is children aged 11–16 years, whose discrete needs in health services have long been recognised (Ministry of Health *op. cit.*). Unless the importance of providing appropriate services for children and young people is recognised and acted upon, inequalities in health between children from different areas and different social class backgrounds are unlikely to be addressed.

Services designed for children and run by staff qualified in the care of children are generally only to be found in children's hospitals, located in some major cities. Specialist children's services such as paediatric intensive care, bone marrow transplant, head injury treatment, burns treatment and some forms of surgery are increasingly only to be found in children's hospitals. Whilst acknowledging that these centres provide the best care for children they can be hundreds of miles away from the child's home, raising significant questions about inequalities in access. Accommodation is usually provided for at least one carer; the disruption to family life for children and carers living in distant areas can have extensive effects. The emotional, social and financial costs to families whose children are receiving such care, sometimes over long periods of time, have been well recorded (Goulding 1992, Callery 1997). Callery observes that mothers take time off work and often leave their jobs in order to be with their children, causing considerable personal stress as they try to care for their sick child and continue to manage the family from afar on a reduced budget.

It is interesting to note Denny's observations in Chapter Four of this volume concerning the development of children's nursing. Historically the role of the children's nurse was equated with the caring role of a nanny and therefore not considered suitable for the middle classes. The development of nursing specialisms was influenced by class divisions within the profession and by class differences in views about women's work. Nursing children, whether as the children's nurse, health visitor or school nurse are all professions traditionally strongly associated with women. Hence the status of children's nursing is particularly closely linked to the status of women as well as that of children. Today working with children remains predominantly women's work. Of the University of the West of England's 2001 intake of students admitted to BSc/Diploma in Children's Nursing courses, only five per cent were male. The percentage of men on other nursing programmes is at least ten per cent. Until fairly recently children's nurse education was even considered by some to be an excellent preparation for 'those nurses who chose to leave for marriage and a family of their own' (Duncombe and Weller 1971: vi).

The role of children's nurses in the 21st century

School nurses

Despite recognition that the health care of the nation's children requires much more than a maternal role there is overwhelming evidence that specialist children's nursing services, for example school nursing and community children's nursing, are not meeting current need. School nursing has long been a 'Cinderella service' of the nursing profession. They have received inadequate training opportunities and low status with accompanying poor career progression for many years and in some areas school nurses have experienced the complete removal of the service altogether. Historically, school nurses have each worked in only one school, providing a public health role as well as a screening service and first aid. Today school nurses frequently have a caseload of 2000–2500 children attending a range of primary, secondary and special schools. Working part time and in term time only, the role of the school nurse has been particularly attractive to mothers of school age children and those returning to nursing. No extra training has been deemed necessary and indeed applicants do not have to be children's nurses. Their main role has been to provide developmental screening and health promotion, although different areas have different priorities. The priorities can place school nurses under particular pressure when there are threats to the public health. In order to carry out Government led mass immunisation campaigns, notably against measles, mumps and rubella (MMR) in 1997 and meningitis C in 2001, for example, school nurses have had to reschedule and cancel large amounts of health promotion activity. Such campaigns have left school nurses feeling frustrated at the need to respond to political priorities and not necessarily the health needs of local children. They have subsequently questioned the value attributed to their health promotion role.

The Labour government's public health White Paper, *Saving Lives: Our Healthier Nation* (DoH 1999c), identifies school nurses as key workers in working with school aged children, especially on health promotion and mental health issues; however until recently this role has not been fully recognised and has consequently been under-resourced. Some areas are now reviewing the practice of school nurses, especially as regards screening programmes, and enhancing the public health role of their practitioners (DeBell and Jackson 2000). The development of the school nurse's role in public health, however, has been hampered by a prolonged lack of interest in the health needs of primary school aged children. Children between the ages of five and eleven years have not been a popular subject for research and discussion. There is little published work on this age group. Most authors prefer to concentrate on the under fives or on young people at secondary school, the latter being an age group which provides a wealth of rich material for health writers including, for example, on drugs and alcohol and sex education. Salmon and Watson (2000) in a scoping survey of health visitors, school nurses and midwives found that very few parenting education activities provided by these professionals were aimed at children aged five to ten years. Other writers have found that children in this age group could benefit from specific health interventions. The Pyramid Trust (2002), for example, works with nine year olds to improve self esteem as part of a strategy attempting to prevent depression in adulthood.

Health visitors

Health visitors have developed as a professional group with a growing responsibility for parenting, child health and health promotion. *Saving Lives: Our Healthier Nation* encourages health visitors to 'develop a family centred public health role, working with individuals, families and communities to improve health and tackle health inequality' (DoH *op. cit.*: Section 11.6). Health visitors are identified as the leaders of teams which will provide, among other activities, child health programmes, parenting support and education, and advice on family relationships and support to vulnerable children and their families. Members of the team could be nurses, nursery nurses and community workers. This is a considerable challenge for health visitors who, like school nurses, have not necessarily received educational preparation for leadership roles in multidisciplinary teams, nor, indeed, for an understanding of the importance of the child centred approach adopted by children's nurses. Health visiting has a very different history from children's nursing and entry to health visiting has traditionally been restricted to adult or general trained nurses. In primary health care, the assumed superiority of general nurse training, discussed in Chapter Four, is exemplified through the assumed leadership status of health visiting. The historical legacy of class differences within nursing may be influencing nurses' collective ability to work together to provide health services which can address health inequalities through meeting the needs of all children and their families.

Recognition of the difficulties many separate professional groups across health and social care have in working together may have contributed to the Labour government's decision to establish an interdepartmental initiative to promote the health and wellbeing of families and young children before and from birth. The Sure Start programme, which began in 1999, aims to work with parents-to-be, parents and children to promote the physical, intellectual and social development of babies and young children — particularly those who are disadvantaged — so that they can flourish at home and when they get to school, and thereby break the cycle of disadvantage for the current generation of young children (Sure Start website www.surestart.gov.uk).

Health visitors are the professional group particularly likely to be involved in Sure Start initiatives in local areas, but some programmes around Britain have the potential to link a range of professional services supporting child health. In the South West, the North Prospect LARK Project, for example, offers the services of a community paediatrician and a child psychologist to support the health of young children. Health visitors work alongside a range of workers supporting family health through support for adults, welfare benefits advice, youth services, and support for families with behavioural needs. The development of nurses' skills in community work and partnership working are particular challenges.

Community children's nursing

The one area that child health professionals agree is the most inequitable in children's nursing is children's community nursing (CCN). Historically and today the vast majority of sick children are cared for at home, usually by their mothers. Perhaps because this care has been taken for granted a universal children's community nursing service has not been deemed necessary. The inadequacy in national provision severely restricts children's nurses' ability to participate in family centred approaches to developing public health, such as the Sure Start initiatives.

The establishment of the current children's community nursing service, such as it is, appears to have arisen to meet local need and therefore represents many different models of provision. Whiting (2000) describes such models:

- using the district nursing service by 'converting' some district nurses to children's nurses, allowing them to care for adults and children
- creating a specific CCN service based in the local hospital, giving the practitioners the opportunity to follow children from the acute to the primary sectors and thus provide a seamless service
- a CCN service based on a medical model with specialist community children's nurses caring for children with a specific condition. The CLIC (Cancer and Leukaemia in Children) nurses are a good example of these practitioners, with many of these nurses and the service they provide being funded by the charity
- other specialist nurses work for medical teams, with the role being created by the relevant consultant in charge to care for 'their' patients.

Whiting suggests that the variety of different models of CCN service is meeting the needs of sick children at home and that a variety of provision will continue to emerge. The specialist model has been criticised where it exists as the only service. It is argued that a specialist service fails to meet the needs of a large number of sick children who do not have a discrete diagnosis and those children with multiple health problems. There is also an issue of 'ownership' with children and their families being cared for by specialists by virtue of their condition. Other children with similar needs, but a different condition, may be excluded from the service.

In areas where there are no children's community nurses, children and their families can receive care from a variety of practitioners who do not have specialist knowledge of caring for children. Families in this situation complain of confusion and frustration as practitioners are unable to supply them with relevant support and information (Health Committee 1997). Other families receive no support or elect to manage by themselves. Families in these circumstances rely on each other as well as friends and neighbours, resulting in high stress levels, mental health problems and frequent incidents of relationship breakdown. Parents rely on well children in the family to care for the sick child and to support their parents by shopping, washing and cooking, leaving these 'young carers' deprived of appropriate social interactions and educational opportunities (Hutt 2000).

In 1959, Platt recommended that there should be a rapid increase in the children's community nursing service to support and care for the thousands of sick children at home (Ministry of Health *op. cit.*). In 2000, 50 per cent of the country was still without such a service (Muir and Sidey *op. cit.*). As such a service is available to the adult population by way of the district nursing service, surely the children of this country deserve equal provision. Fradd, writing in the foreword to Muir and Sidey (*op. cit.*: xvii) concurs: 'Equitable services ensure the right of any child to be offered care whatever their circumstances.'

The future

Children have fewer chances to access equal opportunities legislation than the rest of the population and lack the political power of adults to lobby for improvements in services pertinent to them. The call for a minister for children or an equivalent representative to act as an advocate in issues relevant to children, as suggested by the Kennedy Report (Kennedy *op. cit.*) has so far met with little consideration in England but has found support in Scotland and Wales. In 1989 the United Nations published the International Convention on the Rights of the Child (ratified by the United Kingdom in 1991) advocating that children have a right to be cared for in child centred services (Newell 1991). Child health services have made great improvements in attempting to achieve this goal in the last thirteen years; however there is still a long way to go.

One of the challenges for children's nurses is how to develop their own role as child centred specialists within multiprofessional teams which have a responsibility to consider the broader interests of families and communities. An understanding of the social context of child health illuminates patterns of inequality and may help improve services for the most disadvantaged children. Developing child centred services to meet diverse local needs will play an important role in promoting health for the next generation.

8 Income and health: implications for community nursing

Robert Hoskins

Introduction

The relationship between income and health is not new. We know that the higher an individual's income is, the better their health will be. What is new however are theories that have tried to shed light on how income affects health. This chapter introduces the reader to the importance of income as a determinant of health by examining the claims of three competing theories: the relative income theory (Wilkinson 1996a); the individual/absolute income theory; and the neomaterialism theory (Shaw *et al.* 1999), which describe conflicting mechanisms as to how income impacts on health.

New Labour's rediscovery of poverty and a commitment to tackle health inequalities will also be critically examined. Attention will then focus on the potential of nurses to boost the incomes of their frail clients by accessing the untapped reserve of £2.5–4bn of welfare benefits which lie unclaimed every year in Britain (Davis 2000). The unique attributes of primary care as an arena for nurses to maximise the incomes of their most vulnerable clients by means of welfare benefit screening will also be critically examined.

Finally, an innovative approach to welfare benefit screening involving community nurses screening the frail elderly for unclaimed attendance allowance will also be examined.

I am sure every community nurse who has patients who live in deprived and affluent areas has often asked themselves: why is it that more affluent patients live to a ripe old age in contrast to those who come from more economically deprived backgrounds? The following section of this chapter will address this question by looking at an important component of poverty, which is lack of income and its effects on health. We will now look at the three competing theories that attempt to explain how income impacts on health.

The relative income theory

This theory suggests that in countries which have experienced the increase in life expectancy associated with the transition from an underdeveloped to a developed modern economy, it is not how rich a country is in terms of absolute income as measured by gross domestic product (GDP) that is the key to health, but how equitably that income is distributed that counts (Wilkinson 1992). Evidence from Taiwan, a country that has recently made the epidemiological transition associated with the move from an underdeveloped to a modern economy, suggests that the relationship between income inequality and health had become much stronger by 1999 when the economy had matured than in 1976 when it was still developing. Chiang (1999) concludes that the health of the Taiwanese population was affected more by relative income than by absolute income as a result of the change from a developing to a modern economy.

Further evidence in support of this theory cites the USA as being the richest country in the world in terms of GDP but lying 20th in the world ranking for life expectancy behind poorer countries such as Costa Rica (Kawachi *et al.* 1999).

Life expectancy and income distribution

Relative income theorists would argue that another example of the importance of the effects of income distribution on health can be seen in the dramatic contrast in mortality outcomes between Great Britain and Japan between the mid 1970s and 1986. In the mid 1970s both countries had similar life expectancies and similar income distributions, but by 1986 the increase in life expectancy in Japan was the highest in the world, equivalent to the gain in Britain that would have materialised if all British deaths from coronary heart disease and most cancers had been eliminated (Marmot and Davey Smith 1989). What factors could have caused such an improvement in Japanese life expectancy? Wilkinson argues that the answer lies in the divergent economic experiments that both countries embarked upon during the 1980s. Marmot and Davey Smith (*ibid.*) suggest that at the end of the 1980s the Japanese economy had rapidly expanded, creating full employment which resulted in Japan having the narrowest income differentials in the world. This was in marked contrast to Britain where the post-war trend to a more equal society was reversed between 1979 and 1992, which coincided with Margaret Thatcher's leadership of the Conservative government when the real income of the poorest ten per cent of the population fell by 18 per cent, in marked contrast to that of the richest ten per cent which rose by 61 per cent (Oppenheim and Harker 1996). However, recent research would suggest that income inequality in Japan has increased markedly since the late 1980s. A study assessing the effects on self rated health of individual income and income distribution in Japan concluded that individual/ absolute income was more strongly associated with self rated health than income inequality (Shibuya *et al.* 2002).

Income inequality and how it impacts on individual and population health

Wilkinson argues that income inequality translates through perceptions of one's place in the social hierarchy based on rel- ative position according to income (Lynch *et al.* 2000). Adverse position in the social hierarchy, as determined by rel- ative income, impacts within and outwith the individual by means of psychosocial pathways (Wilkinson 1996a). Within the individual, adverse social position causes feelings of shame and distrust leading to chronic stress which translates biolog- ically through neuro-endocrine pathways, weakening the body's immune system, thus making individuals more prone to illness and more prone to taking up unhealthy coping mechanisms such as smoking and alcohol abuse, leading to poorer health (*ibid.*). Outwith the individual, it is these adverse negative biological effects which determine how individuals interact socially with their environment, which can lead to feelings of social exclusion, hostility and antisocial behaviour which can erode civic trust and cause a breakdown in social cohesion and in social capital (*ibid.*). For example, in the 1950s, in spite of similar smoking rates to neighbouring areas, Roseto, a small Italian-American community in Pennsylvania, demonstrated lower death rates from heart attacks than neighbouring communities. Roseto differed from the other towns as it was remarkably close knit, with a strong sense of family and camaraderie where the inhabitants looked out for one another. This led researchers to conclude that this sense of close knit community protected the health of the inhabitants in some way. However, this health advantage eroded during the affluent 1960s when younger people moved away, family ties became looser and people became more concerned with rampant materialism, which in turn led to a rapid widening of income differentials.

If widening income differentials have a negative impact on life expectancy, there is evidence to suggest that narrowing income distribution has a positive impact on population health. Wilkinson (*op. cit.*) cites Winter's (1985, 1988) studies which identified a dramatic increase in life expectancy at birth in the English and Welsh population of between six and seven years during both World Wars. This increase occurred despite health services being geared towards treating war casualties and was twice as fast as the average rate of improvement of any other decade between 1900 and 1990. A variety of factors have been cited as being responsible for this. These factors include a return to full employment, and a narrowing of income differentials between rich and poor, resulting in a unifying effect within the population which promoted social cohesion and longevity, especially in poorer areas.

The individual/absolute income theory

The individual or absolute income hypothesis argues that the less income we as individuals have the less able we are to afford to eat healthily, keep ourselves warm, or afford quality housing. Exponents of this theory would suggest that it is this lack of absolute income to buy essential material goods which impacts negatively on our health. Absolute income theory argues that there is evidence to suggest that among underdeveloped countries there exists a strong relationship between absolute income in terms of gross national product (GNP) and life expectancy: the lower the GNP, the lower the average life expectancy (World Bank 1993). However critics of absolute income theory argue that the relationship between absolute income and life expectancy disappears when per capita income reaches a certain threshold, rendering further increases in GNP as having negligible impact on increasing life expectancy (Wilkinson *op. cit.*).

Supporters of the individual income theory argue that the relationship of income to health at the individual level is important in understanding health differences between individuals in developed economies (Lynch *et al. op. cit.*). Unlike exponents of the relative income theory, the individual income interpretation assumes that the determinants of population health are not related to how equitably income is distributed within a population but instead are related to the independent health attributes of individuals within a population. This theory suggests that the health effects seen at the population level are a reflection of the sum total of individual effects (Diez-Roux 1998, Koopman and Lynch 1999). A recent study of the subject reinforces this point and found that the effect that income inequality (relative income) had on life expectancy in Denmark disappeared after adjustment for individual income and other factors (Osler *et al.* 2002). It is interesting to note, that in contrast to the findings of Koopman and Lynch (1999), Diez-Roux (1998) and Osler *et al.* (2002), who noted that the relationship between relative income and health disappeared after adjustment for individual income, Wolfson *et al.* (1999) defend the relative income explanation. They conclude, in an income distribution study based on 1990 data for US states, that the strength of observed levels of association between income inequality and mortality may go well beyond what can be explained as a statistical artefact of an individual level relation between income and mortality.

Despite much observational literature linking income to health there appears to be an absence of randomised controlled studies which have assessed the potential for income supplementation to be used to improve health (Connor *et al.* 1999). One exception to this is the following study by Kehrer and Wolin (1979) which looked at pregnancy as an outcome measure. This study was carried out on two groups of pregnant women in Gary, Indiana, USA between 1970 and 1974. The intervention group received an expanded income support plan that guaranteed a minimum income to a group of mothers with low income. Mothers at high risk of adverse pregnancy outcome had heavier babies if they had received the income support plan (*ibid.*).

The neomaterialism theory

Neomaterialism is a term used to both differentiate this theory from, and link it to, Marx's materialist theory of history. Exponents of this theory indict poverty and not income inequality as the most plausible causal explanation for health inequalities. Neomaterialists have been the most vociferous of critics of the psychosocial explanation of health inequalities, suggesting instead that health inequalities are caused by the cumulative effects of poverty over the life course (from conception to death) and not by the psychosocial effects of one's relative position in the social hierarchy at one point in time. What appears to be important is not any one factor which has a major long term influence on health, but a number of comparatively small differences which become linked to a chain of disadvantage (Blane 1999). Bartley *et al.* (1997) argue that in the absence of suitable resources, the accumulation of negative material factors in early life such as poor foetal development, low birth weight, and poor educational attainment ultimately damage health and inevitably lead to a life trajectory of further disadvantage.

Neomaterialism theory would not only see income inequality as but one manifestation of a cluster of neomaterial conditions that affect population health but also would cite the individual income hypothesis plus neomaterialism theory as providing a better fit with the available evidence (Lynch *et al. op. cit.*). Under a neomaterialist interpretation, unequal income distribution affects health at the individual level by a combination of negative exposure throughout the life course, which can affect individual purchasing of material essentials such as food and housing, and by income inequality leading to underinvestment in vital public services which impact on health throughout the life course (*ibid.*).

Discussion

Of the three theories that have attempted to explain how income impacts on life expectancy, the one that has been most critically appraised of all is the relative income theory. Different aspects of the relative income theory have recently been subjected to a barrage of sustained criticism. Some critics suggest that the empirical evidence in support of this theory is methodologically flawed (Judge 1995, Lynch *et al. op. cit.*), suggesting that Wilkinson was selective with the countries that he chose in his seminal 1992 article to show the relationship between income distribution and life expectancy. Lynch *et al.* (*ibid.*) revisited Wilkinson's initial dataset, expanded it by including all countries where gross domestic product was greater than $10,000 per head, and found a statistically significant relationship between absolute income (GDP) and life expectancy ($p > 0.003$), suggesting that the association between absolute income and health hinges on which wealthier countries are examined.

A more recent study (Lynch *et al.* 2001) using better quality data also shows no association between life expectancy and income inequality within 16 Western industrialised countries, apart from a strong relationship to infant mortality. Lynch and colleagues conclude that 'Income inequality and characteristics of the psychosocial environment like trust, control, and organisational membership do not seem to be key factors in understanding health differences between these wealthy countries.' The only country left which now replicates Wilkinson's original proposed relationship between income inequality and life expectancy is the USA (Kaplan *et al.* 1996, Kennedy *et al.* 1996).

Wilkinson's psychosocial pathways explanation as to how income inequality impacts at an individual level by means of a person's relative position in a social hierarchy has also been criticised for relying too heavily on primate studies to explain the physiological effects of adverse hierarchical position on humans (Davey Smith 1996). Lynch *et al.* (*op. cit.*) have also criticised Wilkinson's conceptualisation of social cohesion and social capital as being superficial, as this ignores the crucial impact exerted by political, economic and legal structures. Critics of the income inequality theory, especially the neomaterialists, also argue that its evidence base has been gathered from cross-sectional surveys which provide a snapshot of income distribution at one time point only. Neomaterialists would argue that cross-sectional studies are unable to shed much light on causal effects as they miss crucial data gathered throughout the life course and are therefore of little help in shaping policies to reduce health inequalities (Judge and Paterson 2001).

This is a relatively new field of research, indeed it is in its infancy. There has been and continues to be an explosion of articles which are looking at how poverty and income impact on population health. At the moment, the evidence would favour the absolute income theory plus neomaterialism as a more credible explanation as to what causes health inequalities (Lynch *et al. op. cit.*). However, it could also be argued that both relative poverty and neomaterialism theory fail to provide rounded explanations of how health inequalities arise, as the relative income theory underplays the importance of material factors whilst neomaterialism has little to say about how psychosocial factors impact on health. There is some common ground between the two as well, as neomaterialists also accept that increasing income inequality is bad for health in both the short and long term (Davey Smith *op. cit.*), although they would refute the psychosocial explanation of this, suggesting instead that redistributing income will have a positive effect on health due to boosting individual incomes (Lynch and Davey Smith 2002). The solutions of both theories to tackling health inequalities also emphasise the importance of reducing income inequality, although neomaterialism goes further by arguing for the alleviation of poverty through the reduction of inequalities not just in income but also in wealth (Shaw *et al. op. cit.*).

Implications for community nurse practice

Nurses do not have the power to take control of the commanding heights of the economy and redistribute income and narrow the wealth gap; but they do have the potential to boost the incomes of their most disadvantaged clients by screening them for unclaimed welfare benefits, a subject that will be discussed in more detail later in this chapter. Apart from welfare benefit screening, what are the other implications for community nurse practice of the relative income and neomaterialism theories? Of the two, relative income theory would appear to offer community nurses more scope for health promotion practice. Relative income theory argues that the negative effects of income inequality on social hierarchy are mediated through psychosocial pathways, causing chronic stress at an individual level and a withering of community relations and social cohesion at a community level. Nurses have a major role to play in promoting social inclusion. At an individual level, community nurses should be vigilant in supporting socially excluded individuals and families, by means of offering counselling, or referring to an appropriate agency or support group. If nurses are to contribute to promoting social cohesion in disadvantaged communities they need to rediscover their public health role. The RCN (1994) suggests six public health nursing activities (please see Box 8.1) that community nurses can use in deprived areas to promote social capital — the invisible glue that binds a healthy society together.

If relative income theory offers community nurse practice the potential for intervention at both the individual and community levels, what implications does neomaterialism theory have for community nursing?

Neomaterialism theory advocates that government interventions that reduce health inequalities should be targeted at crucial times throughout the life course (Bartley *et al. op cit.*). Box 8.2 identifies these critical periods during the life course where individuals are at their most vulnerable and susceptible to ill health due to an accumulation of material disadvantage. The 'knock on' consequences of cumulative material disadvantage have major implications for community nurse practice and can be demonstrated as follows. Poor nutrition and poor

---

Box 8.1 Key activities for public health nursing

- Assess the health needs of local populations through the compilation of health profiles
- Support people to participate in the life of their community to influence factors that affect their health
- Increase health resources in communities by establishing local networks
- Build healthy alliances and a supportive infrastructure to provide information, resources and practical help for community initiatives
- Engage with the local statutory and voluntary groups to work towards health related policies and actions
- Increase uptake of health services by ensuring they are accessible, offered appropriately and effectively targeted

Source: Royal College of Nursing (1994)

Box 8.2 Critical periods of the life course

- Foetal development
- Birth
- Nutrition, growth and health in childhood
- Educational career
- Leaving parental home
- Establishing social and sexual relationships
- Job loss or insecurity
- Parenthood
- Episodes of illness
- Labour market exit
- Loss of full independence

Source: Shaw *et al.* (1999), adapted from Bartley *et al.* (1997)

---

maternal environment can cause the developing foetus to be born thin, with low birth weight (Barker 1995). Thin underweight infants are disadvantaged by being more prone to coronary heart disease in later life (Eriksson *et al.* 2001). Therefore, it is precisely at this critical period during the life course that nurses need to offer their pregnant clients extra support to stop smoking, reduce alcohol and follow a healthy diet. Nurses also need to encourage pregnant clients who live in deprived areas to participate in new Government initiatives such as Sure Start. The Sure Start programme is geared specifically to promoting a healthy pregnancy and breaking the cycle of disadvantage for the current generation of young children by encouraging the physical, social and intellectual development of babies and youngsters (Sure Start 2002).

It is important not to forget that the renaissance of the public health movement and the health inequalities debate have been greatly influenced by New Labour's commitment to tackling the causes of poverty. The next section will now review the government's track record on this.

New Labour's response to reducing income inequality and tackling health inequalities

It is interesting to note that the Independent Inquiry into Inequalities in Health (Acheson 1998) acknowledged that available evidence on income inequality is insufficient to confirm or deny a causal relationship between changes in income distribution and the parallel deterioration in health inequalities. However, the Inquiry's report also took the view that these changes are likely to be related and stated that *crucial* steps should be taken to reduce income inequalities to improve the living standards of the poor (*ibid.*). Five years on since the report's publication, how successful has New Labour been in reducing income inequality? Before one can objectively answer this question one has to take into consideration the extent of the widening health and income gap that New Labour inherited when first coming to office in 1997. In the 20 years before New Labour came to power, the differences in mortality across social classes widened for both sexes. For example, in the late 1970s, death rates were 53 per cent higher among men in social classes IV and V, compared with those in classes I and II; by the late 1980s, they were 68 per cent higher (*ibid.*).

New Labour's first term performance

One must also take account of the plethora of policy initiatives that Labour has implemented to address this issue in its first term such as the New Deal, the minimum wage, increases in child benefit and the Working Families Tax Credit. It is widely anticipated that these initiatives, which yet have to bear fruit, will increase the economic status of the least well off. However, the latest evidence would suggest that not only has there been a widening of income inequality under New Labour but it has also surpassed the highest inequality mark (1991) which was achieved under the previous successive Conservative governments. The Gini coefficient, which measures the gap in incomes after tax between rich and poor, has risen to 40 on a scale where zero represents universal equality of income; it was 38 in 1997 and increased again to 39 in 1998/99 (Office for National Statistics 2001b). When asked to comment in an interview as to whether he felt that the widening income gap was acceptable, Tony Blair repeatedly refused to answer the question but did say that increasing the basic rate of income tax on the salaries of millionaires was not on his second term agenda. In this one statement he appeared not only to have sacrificed the plight of the poor on the high altar of the free market but also to ride roughshod over the most crucial of all recommendations of the Independent Inquiry, that of reducing income inequalities (Hoskins 2001). He also appeared to jettison his own personal commitment to greater equality made when in opposition where he wrote 'I believe in greater equality. If the next Labour Government has not raised the living standards of the poorest by the end of its time in office it will have failed' (quoted in Howarth *et al.* 1998: 9).

The legacy of the Blair government's first term attempt to tackle poverty is mixed and comprised of an adherence to Conservative spending plans for the first two years of office; a widening income divide and child poverty figures which fell by only 500,000, well short of the 1.2 million claimed by the government (Child Poverty Action Group 2001). Will New Labour's second term mark an improvement?

New Labour's second term performance

It would appear that New Labour's second term is far more fiscally adventurous than previously. Free from the shackles of the self-imposed state spending restrictions of their first two years in office, 2002 saw New Labour return to its Old Labour 'high tax and spend' instincts, with two massive public spending pledges. Firstly, the 2002 Budget saw the government commit itself to an extra £40bn of investment in the NHS over five years, which will increase NHS funding from the current £65bn to £103bn in 2007/8, funded from a 1p in the pound increase in National Insurance payments. Secondly, an additional £61bn is being invested in public services such as education, transport and child care over a three year period.

It would therefore appear that New Labour is waging a full frontal fiscal assault on the causes of poverty by investing heavily in public services and is also providing a sustained attempt at redistribution as well. For example, in the first term we had a strict adherence to tackling redistribution by increasing stealth taxes such as petrol tax and promoting equality of opportunity through the New Deal and the minimum wage. However, we now see a massive investment being made in public services and the promotion of equality of outcome through increasing National Insurance contributions, with the hint that an increase in income tax might also occur. It would appear that New Labour has now realised that the actions of the Chancellor of the Exchequer have far more potential to improve the health of the nation than those of the Secretary of State for Health (Quick and Wilkinson 1991).

Welfare benefits screening as a means of reducing income inequality

However, there is another major economic lever that the Government could also pull that has the potential to improve the economic status of thousands of chronically sick people in Britain. The Independent Inquiry report also urged the government to take action to increase the uptake of welfare benefits by entitled groups (Acheson *op. cit.*). Due to the fraudulent activity of a few, the media coverage associated with welfare benefit recipients inevitably tends to be negative, highlighting stories about benefit fraud. However, the reality is the opposite from the adverse media portrayal as the amount of money that goes unclaimed on income support alone every year exceeds the amount which is paid out on fraudulent claims. More than £2bn is stolen in benefits fraud in the UK every year (Department of Work and Pensions 2002); however this sum is more than equalled by the £2.02–£4.2bn of means tested benefit that went unclaimed in the UK in 1998/99 (Davis 2000). The DSS (1989) estimated that 33 per cent of pensioners (around one million) who were entitled to income support and 18 per cent who were entitled to housing benefit did not claim it. Results from the Family Resources Study also identified the fact that only 40–60 per cent of eligible pensioners were taking up attendance allowance (Craig and Greenslade 1998).

Over the last 10–15 years there has been considerable interest in exploring the most effective way of getting this money out to its rightful recipients. One of the most potentially effective methods of accessing the traditional under-claimer is in the primary care setting. The following sub-section draws on Hoskins' and Carter's (2000) review of the literature, which not only examines the advantages that primary care holds as an arena for maximising income but it also looks at the potential of the community nurse to become a major player in this new field.

Primary care as an arena for welfare benefits screening

There would appear to be strong evidence that would endorse situating a welfare benefit uptake project in primary care. Hobby *et al.* (1998) cite Galvin's arguments that primary care welfare benefits projects give vital access to money advice to marginalised groups who might otherwise be excluded from this service through lack of transport, being too ill, too poor or too old. Paris and Player (1993) argue that situating benefit uptake projects in primary care settings introduces money advice to a totally different audience from the one that visits a Citizens' Advice Bureau (CAB). Ennals (1990: 1321) argues that there is a unique natural linkage between welfare benefit uptake and primary care workers as health care workers provide evidence in support of certain claims such as attendance allowance, disability living allowance and incapacity benefit.

This finding was also endorsed by Middleton *et al.* (1993), who found that the average number of welfare benefit officer contacts per patient who attended a health centre was much higher than for those patients who were contacted by the same welfare benefits officer outwith a primary care setting. The authors also argue that the health centre patients had more complex problems in comparison to those patients seen outwith the health centre setting.

Paris and Player (*op. cit.*) uncovered £58,000 of unclaimed benefit for 39 clients, of which £54,000 was annually recurring, by placing a CAB worker to cover sessions in several GP practices in Birmingham over a three month period. Middleton *et al.* (*op. cit.*) identified £24,751 for 18 clients, £10,393 of which was in the form of lump sums and £14,358 recurring on an annual basis, by placing a welfare benefits adviser for two hour and a half sessions a week over a six month period in a health centre. An expanded version of this project which ran for six months in four GP surgeries and included employing two full time equivalent welfare rights advisers raised £20,933 of unclaimed benefit, 60 per cent of which was in the form of lump sum payments and 40 per cent was continuing income. Veitch (1995) identified 28 clients who together were entitled to £1,423 per week on an annualised basis plus a one off lump sum of £28,784 during a pilot welfare benefit uptake project located in two Birmingham health centres. Some £1,334,142 of unclaimed benefits were raised between 1992 and 1997, of which £404,800 were identified in 1996/97 by three CAB workers providing 43 hours of benefits advice for 12 health centres per week (North Tyneside Citizens' Advice Bureau 1997). Some £323,000 of unclaimed benefit were raised for 157 people over a six month pilot period in a health centre project in Islington which featured money advice training for primary care staff, plus welfare benefits worker input (Griffiths 1992). Over a two year period the North Derbyshire 'Welfare Rights in Primary Care' project identified £1,292,406 of annualised benefits in the years 1996 and 1998 (North Derbyshire RDA Project 1998). A Glasgow medical centre ran a money and benefits advice service staffed by a money advice worker in two general practices and recovered £66,785 in the initial setup year for 42 patients (Cornwallis and O'Neil 1998).

Is there a role for community nurses in this area?

There is a debate to be had as to whether community nurses should screen their frail clients for unclaimed welfare benefits. Some might argue whether that is the job of the social services and not that of nursing. Perhaps one could have justified that response before the election of a government committed to tackling health inequalities. However, the White Paper, *Towards a Healthier Scotland* (Scottish Office Department of Health 1999) has recognised that if health inequalities are going to be reduced it will take a collective effort on the part of society to do this, and that most importantly includes nurses. In fact *Towards a Healthier Scotland* not only recognised nurses' potential as being major players in tackling health inequalities, it also recognised that nurses had to work in new ways to achieve this new role and instructed the Chief Nursing Officer to review the public health role of the community nurse (Scottish Executive 2001). The RCN has recently encouraged nurses to become active in welfare benefit screening as a means of reducing the health gap (Nursing Times 1999). The RCN (1996) also suggests that community nurses are already screening their clients for unclaimed benefits and they recommend as well that welfare benefit work should become a major component of health profiling where the claiming of means tested welfare benefits is a good indicator of poverty.

There are other ways that community nurses can encourage income maximisation. Community nurses are now encouraged to work with others to tackle health inequalities in the new NHS structures such as Health Action Zones (England and Wales), Primary Care Trusts (England and Wales), Local Health Care Cooperatives and New Community Schools (Scotland). These new structures allow community nurses access to influence the delivery of health care and health promotion services by arguing for welfare benefit uptake projects to be placed high on the purchasing agenda (Hoskins 1999). An admission to hospital for some patients often leads to a major change in future quality of life due to incapacity. Therefore, hospital nurses have a major role to play in ensuring that patients who fall into this category are either seen by a social worker for a benefits appraisal whilst they are still in hospital or in arranging for a benefits assessment when they are back in the community as part of patient discharge planning.

For those community nurses who wish to respond to the spirit of the White Paper and develop a public health role in their work, the RCN (1998) recommends that the health visiting service should become more actively involved in poverty profiling by collecting health information such as receipt of welfare benefits. It would appear that community nurses are in an ideal position to provide this service as they are also trusted by the public and gain intimate knowledge of their clients because of their daily contact in their homes (*ibid.*). This relationship is established at the first visit to a new client which often provides community nurses with an excellent opportunity to collect information on their client's benefit status and refer those who could potentially gain from a more in depth welfare benefits screening to a money advice worker.

The inclusion of welfare benefits screening and referral amongst an extensive repertoire of other health promoting services gives community nurses a unique opportunity to address adverse life circumstances and demonstrate to their clients that they are aware of the link between low income and poor health. Naidoo and Wills (1998) have argued that the provision of a welfare benefits referral service is a useful addition to the health promotion toolbox as it avoids 'victim blaming', by focussing on benefit entitlement and not unhealthy lifestyles.

Blackburn and Graham's (1992) information pack on 'Smoking among working class women', which was designed to influence the health promotion practice of health visitors, practice nurses, midwives and other community nurses, also acknowledges this link. The pack was based on the findings of Graham's (1992) study, which looked at how tobacco was used by mothers in working class households. Blackburn and Graham discovered that women might find it easier to stop smoking and maintain smoking cessation if some of the material stresses associated with smoking and caring for children were also relieved. Their recommendations for health promotion practice reflect this and suggest that community nurses should help women to claim the social security benefits to which they are entitled, as the uptake of benefits that are crucial to women such as family credit is low. They also recommend that nurses should give women benefits information and help them gain access to welfare rights advice and debt counselling services.

Perhaps one of the reasons why there has been so little evidence of community nurse research in this area, in spite of the legitimacy given to it by the RCN, is that so few resources appear to have been developed to encourage nurse involvement in welfare benefits screening. There may be reasons for this. One of the perennial problems surrounding welfare benefits is that benefit information resources and training can quickly become obsolete as the inclusion and exclusion criteria for welfare benefit uptake are prone to alteration from one Budget to the next. This in turn means that training needs are recurrent and community practitioners need to be very knowledgeable about the system, to avoid giving incorrect advice to their clients.

It is also important that welfare benefits resources are kept as simple and easy to use as possible, as GPs and community nurses are not equipped to guide patients through the state benefits system, due in part to ignorance of the complex inclusion and exclusion criteria (Jarman 1985). Perhaps lessons could be learned from the community nurses who were involved in the Wigan and Leigh 'welfare benefits in primary care' initiative. These nurses stated that they did not want to become skilled in giving out welfare advice to clients; rather they wanted to know when to refer a client for advice and when not to (Reid 1998).

It is very likely that a high proportion of a community nurse's caseload will include the mentally ill, the chronically sick (Veitch *op. cit.*), the elderly, the low income family and ethnic minorities, all of whom have a history of not claiming benefits to which they are entitled (Oppenheim and Harker *op. cit.*). The community nurse is therefore ideally placed to not only identify the benefit status of these patients on his/her caseload, but more importantly to refer all clients who are believed to be under-claiming to a benefits advice worker for a more in depth 'financial makeover'.

Incapacity benefit, disability living allowance and attendance allowance are directly related to ill health and disability and are the health related benefits with whose potential recipients nurses are most likely to come into contact with on a daily basis. But which benefit should nurses target and screen for? The two benefits which nurses should concentrate on are disability living allowance for frail clients aged between three and 64, and attendance allowance for the frail elderly aged over 64. Both these benefits are non-contributory, non-income related and non-means tested, which means that they can be claimed on behalf of clients irrespective of their financial status.

Let us take the case of attendance allowance as an example. Attendance allowance is a 'passport' benefit which if awarded can trigger other benefit entitlements such as a higher rate of income support, which means it is a very efficient and effective benefit for nurses to screen for. There are currently two rates of attendance allowance paid out to clients aged over 64 years as a result of an illness or disability which has lasted for at least six months. The low rate of £37.65 is paid weekly, (£1957.80 per year) if the patient has either day or night care needs; the high rate of £56.25 per week (£2925 per year) is paid weekly if the patient has both day and night care needs. Special rules also apply to clients who are not expected to live for six months, or clients who use a kidney machine at home or in a self care unit two or more times per week.

Community nurse led welfare benefits screening

What is the most effective way for nurses to screen their clients for unclaimed attendance allowance? As attendance allowance is linked to disability, there is evidence to suggest that many eligible pensioners might be on the caseloads of community nurses and might be either unable or unwilling to attend open access citizens' advice sessions due to poor health and/or lack of money. For example, of the £510,324 in unclaimed benefits uncovered by Easterhouse Money Advice Centre (EHMAC) in two GP surgeries in 2001 only £24,000 were in attendance allowances, which would suggest that open access welfare benefits clinics, even when located in GP surgeries, may not suit the needs of the frail elderly under-claimer (EHMAC 2002).

Hoskins and Smith (2002) implemented a nurse led welfare benefits screening study which was conducted in a deprived area in Glasgow. This study used an innovative model of attendance allowance screening which involved community nurses attached to one general practice located in the most unhealthy parliamentary constituency in Britain (Shaw *et al. op. cit.*) using a specially designed attendance allowance screening form (please see Appendix to this chapter). Community nurses used this form to opportunistically screen clients aged over 64 who looked frail. If the form indicated that the client was likely to qualify for unclaimed attendance allowance the nurse sent it to a welfare rights officer who contacted the client by phone and arranged for a home visit to screen not only for unclaimed attendance allowance but for other benefits as well.

Some 86 clients were opportunistically screened by community nurses for unclaimed attendance allowance over a three month period. Of the 69 clients who were referred to the welfare rights officer for a home benefits assessment, 51 had their cases referred to the DSS. Of the 51 DSS referrals, 37 clients plus four relatives received a total of £112,892 of which £95,306 was on a recurrent annualised basis and £17,587 was paid out as lump sums. The maximisation of income for the four relatives was an anticipated bonus of this model as the welfare rights officer not only screened the benefits status of the referred under-claimant but also screened for appropriate other frail family members as well.

The anticipated 'passport' potential of attendance allowance as a trigger to accessing other benefits was also realised by this study as six clients who received attendance allowance were also successful in their claims for income support. If the amount of money identified by this study were extrapolated to the other 137 general practices in deprivation category 6–7 located in Glasgow, it is envisaged that 2645 frail elderly would together be £7,281,407 better off. More importantly, £6,146,964 would be paid out to them annually (Hoskins and Smith *op. cit.*). The results of this study in terms of amount of benefit successfully claimed within the three month pilot period (£112,892 for 41 clients, £95,306 of which were on a recurrent annualised basis) compares very favourably indeed to the £58,000 uncovered for 39 clients, with £54,000 recurrent annually, reported by Paris and Player (*op. cit.*).

Does a welfare benefit payout boost health?

The Hoskins and Smith (*op. cit.*) study did not attempt to
identify the impact of a welfare benefit payout on the health of
its recipients. Only two studies have been undertaken in primary care that have attempted to identify this (Veitch *op. cit.*,
Abbot and Hobby 1998). Veitch, using a Nottingham Health
Profile, identified positive trends in all areas of health (energy,
sleep and pain levels, emotional reactions, social isolation and
physical mobility) among those who received benefit. Abbot
and Hobby, using an SF36 health profile, identified statistically significant improvements in vitality ($p = 0.002$); role
functioning; emotional ($p = 0.037$) and mental health
($p = 0.005$) among participants who received an income boost
in contrast to those who did not receive additional money.
These statistically significant findings were present at six
months after benefit payout and began to wear off after
12 months, although the 12 month scores were higher than at
first interview (Abbot and Hobby *op. cit.*). Obviously more
rigorous and robust studies in this area are required to identify what, if any, are the precise health benefits of a welfare
benefit payout. However, these initial findings do suggest that
there appears to be an initial 'honeymoon effect' where the
favourable impact on perceived mental health status is
strongest, which dissipates after six months. This window of
opportunity could be maximised by community nurses in
order to bolt on other health promoting initiatives during this
time, which might prolong this perceived improvement in
health status.

Conclusion

It could be argued that the resurgence of interest in the effects
of poverty in generating health inequalities has been fuelled by
a vibrant public health research base, which has in turn gone
some way to shape government policy as to how best to tackle
the problem and reduce its devastating impact on population
health. The research on income and health is an example of
this, whereby the Independent Inquiry (Acheson *op. cit.*) recommended that the government should set out to reduce

income inequalities. The income gap actually widened during New Labour's first term in office, but there are signs that this might be rectified due to a more fiscally adventurous second term. It is only by understanding how poverty impacts on health and the role that lack of income plays in this, that nurses can address this issue with their clients. One explanation as to how lack of income impacts on health is through low relative income and chronic stress at an individual level which erodes community social capital. An alternative mechanism could be through an accumulation of material disadvantage over the life course, either through low absolute income or through a wider range of factors (neomaterialism). Irrespective of which explanation one takes, all theories have important implications for nurse practice in terms of implementing the RCN's six public heath nursing activities (Box 8.1) and intervening to support clients during critical periods during the life course (Box 8.2).

Common to all theories is the importance of reducing income inequality. Neomaterialists reject the psycho-social explanation of the relative income hypothesis but accept that redistributing income will have a positive effect on health due to alleviating poverty through boosting individual incomes (Lynch and Davey Smith 2002). Recent research suggests that nurses have a major role to play in this and can boost the incomes of their frail elderly clients by addressing the Independent Inquiry's recommendation of implementing initiatives which increase welfare benefit uptake, such as screening all frail clients aged 64 and over on their caseloads for unclaimed attendance allowance (Hoskins and Smith *op. cit.*).

Appendix

Community Nurse Attendance Allowance Screening Form

Attendance allowance is for people aged 64 or over who require help with personal care due to illness or disability

Section 1 Is your client currently in receipt of Attendance Allowance?
YES ☐   **NO** ☐   **DON'T KNOW** ☐

If 'yes', which rate of Attendance Allowance is your client currently receiving?
Low rate (£37.65 per week) ☐   **High rate (£56.25 per week)** ☐

Is your client currently in receipt of Disability Living Allowance?
YES ☐   **NO** ☐   **DON'T KNOW** ☐

Please list any health problems/disabilities that your client suffers from:

```



```

Section 2 From your own observations and the client's responses please complete all questions

At any time during the day/night for whatever reason do you feel light headed or dizzy?
YES ☐   **NO** ☐

At any time during the day do you feel pain or severe discomfort when doing normal tasks?
YES ☐   **NO** ☐

During the day/night do you ever feel breathless or get a tightness or pain across your chest?
YES ☐   **NO** ☐

Do you have any serious problems with eyesight/hearing?
YES ☐   **NO** ☐

Do you have any problems caused by your health that mean you require help with everyday tasks?
YES ☐   **NO** ☐

Do you have any recurring problems with your bladder/bowels?
YES ☐   **NO** ☐

Even if the client has answered 'no' to all the questions do you still feel they are needing a lot of assistance?
YES ☐ NO ☐

Does your client have a friend or relative (carer) who assists them with anything, such as bathing, shopping, dressing?
YES ☐ NO ☐

If you have ticked 1 or more 'yes' boxes in section 2, your client could be entitled to AA. Please complete the reverse side of this form to arrange for a WRO home visit.

Client's details

Name ....

DOB .... Age .... Sex .... Telephone ....

Address ....

Post Code ... . GP's Name ....

Does your client have a carer?
YES ☐ NO ☐

Referral details

Please highlight your job title (tick appropriate box)
Health   District   Practice
Visitor   Nurse   Nurse

Date of referral ....../....../......

Nurse's signature: .... Date ....

Client's signature:

I agree to the information contained on this form being passed to a Money Advice Worker who will offer to complete a benefit check in my home.

Signed .... Date ....

Please send this form to:

9 Work and occupational health

Margaret Miers

Introduction

Our daily activities can have a significant effect on our physical and mental health. As the Acheson Report notes, 'people are often defined, and define themselves, through what they do for a living' (Acheson 1998: 44). Our occupation brings status and, as earlier chapters have explained, determines our class position. Employment is 'significant in providing purpose, income, social support, structure to life and a means of participating in society' (*ibid.*: 44–5). The effects of perceptions of purpose, of relative and absolute income, of social support and social participation on an individual's wellbeing remain topics of interest and debate. The authors of the Acheson Report acknowledge the health implications of these varied factors through their recommendations in relation to employment and occupational health. They identify four main policy areas to address employment and health issues. These are: ameliorating health damage through unemployment; preventing unemployment through increasing education and training opportunities; removing barriers to employment through, for example, family friendly measures; and improving employment conditions 'and health-enhancing quality of the work environment' (*ibid.*: 45). The Report's recommendations include measures to improve management practices as well as measures to improve opportunities for work. These recommendations demonstrate a holistic view of health and are based on the findings of a range of studies that show a relationship between ill health and an imbalance between demands and control in the work setting (Marmot *et al.* 1997).

This chapter examines the effects of unemployment on health; the effects of working conditions on health; and the implications of working conditions for the health of nurses and other care workers; and explores nurses' opportunities to change the pattern of health inequalities in relation to occupational health. It begins, however, with a summary of different approaches to explaining the relationship between employment and health. This relationship is not new. Social class differences in mortality and morbidity demonstrate the continuing influence of occupation on patterns of health and disease. Drever *et al.* (2000: 20) report that the average number of years of working life lost for social class I (based on mortality data 1991–93) is 27 years per thousand men aged 20–64. For social class V, for the same age group, there are 87 years of working life lost. The wide difference, however, is increased by the large numbers of deaths from accidents and violence amongst young men in the unskilled group. Occupational differences are only part, albeit an important part, of the class mortality picture.

Why and how does employment affect health?

Negative employment experiences with a negative effect on health are identified as lack of control over work conditions; repetitive and hazardous work conditions (Marmot *et al.* 1991, Pantry 1995); and a lack of status in the workplace, leading to low self esteem and employment insecurity (Heaney *et al.* 1994). Employment insecurity is increasing. Brewster *et al.* (1997), in a European study, identified an increase in part time working, self employment and sub-contracting. Positive work experiences with a positive effect on health include skill development (Hackman and Lawler 1971); autonomy (Kohn and Schooler 1973); and a sense of belonging to a significant group of colleagues (House *et al.* 1988).

The differing views about social inequalities discussed in Chapter One provide different approaches to understanding the nature of work and its health implications in the United Kingdom and similar societies. The 'classical' tradition in sociology, that is, the theories of Durkheim, Marx and Weber, provides approaches to the analysis of work that concentrate on the nature of the division of labour, the relationships of production (in Marx's terms, necessarily oppositional and conflictual) and the methods of organising and controlling work to ensure the continued productivity and profitability of capitalist enterprises. Early studies in industrial sociology took a class analysis for granted and examined workers' experience (Beynon 1975) and their attempts to maintain some control over their workplace (Ditton 1977), describing this as resistance (Thompson and Bannon 1985). More recently, industrial and organisational sociologists have explored the development of 'post-Fordist' management practices and ideas designed to maintain control whilst allowing flexibility in the workforce, production and distribution. (For a review of approaches to understanding nursing work in the labour market, see Miers 1999.) Changing fashions in management practices, however, have led to more critical analyses of power at work, often applying Foucault's analysis of disciplinary power (Foucault 1977) to an analysis of workplace surveillance. A postmodern approach to the analysis of work experience emphasises the possibilities for (and struggles of) individuals to sustain and create an identity for themselves (Fox 1999). The uncertainty of employment affects an individual's sense of self, but the decline of the traditional career can bring individuals more opportunities for choice, including choice about how we see ourselves in relation to work (*ibid.*). This postmodern approach, Thompson and Ackroyd (1995) argue, leads to a neglect of more traditional forms of resistance between worker and employee. I have found it helpful to distinguish three broad approaches to the understanding of employment and health. First a neoMarxist, or neomaterialist approach to class and health inequality advocated by, for example, Scambler and Higgs (1999); second a life course approach (Wadsworth 1996, Blane 1999) and third a postmodern emphasis on possibilities for positive work identities, drawing on the work of Fox (*op. cit.*) and Ezzy (2001).

NeoMarxism and occupational health

Scambler and Higgs (*op. cit.*) argue that social class is a relational concept and therefore relationships between classes should not be ignored. Individuals are placed in relation to other individuals with different positions in the social structure. These different positions bring different material rewards and, in work settings, differing degrees of control over one's own and others' work. Workers perceive themselves as controlled by managers and it is managers who control workload demands. For individuals, perceptions of relative deprivation, of injustice in the workplace, of lack of control over the pace of work, are all conditions that have a negative effect on health (see below). Scambler and Higgs (*ibid.*: 289), drawing on Clement and Myles' work, suggest that health inequalities can only be understood in terms of class relations and particularly through an understanding of the 'obdurate character of the relations between' the 'capitalist-executive', the working class and the new and old middle classes. Clement and Myles (1997) argue that the 'capitalist-executives' have real economic and command power over labour, but the responsibility for command over organisational labour is shared with the new middle class, managers who do not themselves have economic power. The executive class makes strategic decisions. The new middle class makes tactical decisions. The 'old middle class' remains largely outside organisational control so its members do not command others' labour and lack economic power but control their own means of production. (Many professionals, including doctors, could be seen as having been part of this 'old middle class'.) The working class have no economic control and are controlled by others in work. For Scambler and Higgs (*op. cit.*), a relational class analysis can help understand the processes whereby work experiences lead to ill health. If relationships of control influence workers' sense of alienation or of job satisfaction, their perceptions of social support at work, and their sense of injustice or perceived value, it is class relationships which are contributing to workplace wellbeing or workplace stress.

The life course approach

Wadsworth, Blane and colleagues advocate a life course approach to understanding health inequalities. Hoskins, in Chapter Eight, has linked this approach to the neomaterialist approach. Both emphasise the importance of material factors in shaping individual experience. Wadsworth (*op. cit.*) argues that early experiences, including those in the womb, build an individual's 'health capital'. There is considerable evidence that 'health capital' is class related. Wadsworth notes that in lower social class families children are more at risk of respiratory diseases, have a poorer diet and are more likely to live in an environment in which smoking is prevalent than children in other classes. Factors linked to health capital are also linked to factors that contribute to cultural capital, such as education. Education brings occupational opportunities, increasing the chance of retaining security of employment. Continuing insecurity of employment can lead to continuing anxiety and to an absence of the psychosocial support often provided through employment. Anxiety can trigger ill health through cardiovascular damage as a result of stress. In addition, unemployment is linked to marital breakdown, and disruption in family life is also linked to adverse health consequences. Hence adverse trends in employment for age cohorts or for groups in particular occupations (such as workers in mining and steel production) may present a threat to health in the form of 'reduced opportunities for pride in work' (*ibid.*: 163). A life course approach allows the complexity of these factors to be taken into account.

Postmodernism

A postmodernist approach to health and occupation suggests that the flexibility of employment opportunities brings chances to redefine self identity. From this perspective it would be mistaken to assume that individuals will be constrained by traditional class factors or a lack of advantage traditionally associated with lower social class. The positive view of the changing nature of work is that the decline of the lifetime career brings more flexibility and more opportunities for individuals to find different work-life balances and 'more space to develop their talents and potentials' (Bradley 1999: 13). Fox (*op. cit.*: 217) presents an optimistic postmodernist view of the relationship between risk, health and work:

> As a perspective, the postmodern view is not intended to challenge the critiques of industrial production as often injurious to the bodies,

minds and spirits of individuals, but to suggest that the becoming of body, mind or spirit needs to be seen as processual. Health and work are constituted in the unfolding lives of individuals with their own agendas: differently formulated, a risk can — in the right circumstances — be an opportunity to become other.

Ezzy (*op. cit.*) is also interested in the possibilities for individuals to create meaningful working lives within a changing world; however he is critical of over-optimism in relation to the consequences of new forms of work organisation. He is particularly critical of what he terms 'engineered culture' — that is, the cultural dimension of workplace change, which emphasises the importance of flexibility, cooperation and autonomy amongst the workforce. He sees engineered culture as producing a narcissistic individualism, a superficial trust and a 'simulacrum of community' (*ibid.*: 632). Nevertheless he can be seen as supporting Fox's optimism about the fluidity of the post-modern world, and the possibilities inherent in a postmodern 'responsibility to otherness' (White 1991). Ezzy (*op. cit.*: 647) develops an argument for a new 'conception of authenticity that recognises both individual creativity and the requirement for the constraints of community responsibility through a respect for "the other"'.

Evidence about relationships between work and health can be viewed differently depending on the different general theories used to explore and understand the social world. Alongside the general approaches of neomaterialism, the life course and postmodernism, more specific theories and models have been used to identify and examine links between employment, unemployment and health.

Unemployment and health

Research studies consistently demonstrate higher rates of physical ill health (Morris *et al.* 1994, Bartley *et al.* 1996, Nylén *et al.* 2001) and psychological ill health (Warr and Jackson 1987, Montgomery *et al.* 1999) amongst men and women who are unemployed. Bartley *et al.* (1999), analysing data from the National Child Development Study (see Chapter Two) found that at age 33, men who had experienced more unemployment had lower body weight, were more likely to smoke and more likely to have a high score indicative of problem drinking (*ibid.*: 89). Nylén *et al.* (*op. cit.*) report on a longitudinal study of all like sexed twins born in Sweden 1926–58. This study shows excess mortality amongst those who experienced a period of unemployment. Women as well as men demonstrated the association between unemployment and mortality, with a 70 per cent increase in risk amongst women ever unemployed. This is significant, as many studies of unemployment and mortality have concentrated on men.

The psychological effects of unemployment have been identified as lower self esteem, increased anxiety, depression and higher rates of self harm and suicide (Moser *et al.* 1984, Bartley 1994). Montgomery *et al.*'s (*op. cit.*) analysis of the 1958 National Child Development cohort study suggests that longer term unemployment damages the mental health of individuals who were healthy prior to the onset of unemployment. Explanations for the relationships between unemployment are varied. Bartley *et al.* (1996: 256–7) identify four theoretical models:

- Unemployment is a direct cause of ill health, through stress, material hardship and behavioural change
- Unemployment is an indicator of more general insecurity and work hazard. Individuals' skills and work histories lead to difficulties in gaining secure employment
- 'Direct selection': ill health may be a cause of unemployment
- 'Indirect selection': intervening variables such as lower levels of educational attainment or social circumstances which limit work opportunities may provide the link between high risk of unemployment and individual factors.

A specific explanation for the relationship between unemployment and poor mental health has been Marie Jahoda's functionalist approach, which argues that employment fulfils five latent psychological functions. These are: providing a time structure to the day; providing social contacts; participation in collective purposes; providing status and identity; and providing regular activity (Jahoda 1982). Sociologists have welcomed this emphasis on the influence of the environment on mental wellbeing but criticise the assumption that all individuals have unchangeable latent psychological needs. As Nordenmark and Strandh (1999: 579) note, 'from a sociological viewpoint, we must be able to incorporate the notion of a changing society and a changing individual'. They welcome Ezzy's (1993) emphasis on the importance of viewing identity as flexible and socially constructed, not determined by material circumstances. Such a perspective allows the possibility that unemployment has different consequences for different individuals, depending on the extent to which the passage into unemployment disrupts or sustains 'strategies used to sustain a positive self-image' (Nordenmark and Strandh *op. cit.*: 580). They argue that employment serves as a resource to satisfy the need for economic resources as well as the psychosocial need for identity, in a society where employment is the norm. They have developed a model which identifies both economic and psychosocial need and can therefore be used to explain 'both the differences in mental well-being among the unemployed and the changes in individual mental well-being during unemployment and upon re-entering employment' (*ibid.*: 593). Nordenmark and Strandh (*ibid.*) have presented evidence from a longitudinal study in Sweden of 3500 unemployed people and demonstrated that those who have, or manage to develop, low economic and psychological need for employment will retain or regain relatively good mental wellbeing.

Unemployment and people with severe mental illness

It is unsurprising, given the relationship between employment and mental health, that people with severe mental illness experience high rates of unemployment. Crowther *et al.* (2001) note estimates of the unemployment rate in the United Kingdom of 61–73 per cent (Meltzer *et al.* 1995) and estimated rates of 75–85 per cent in the United States (Lehman 1995). These high rates indicate the extent to which those with mental illness experience social exclusion. Crowther *et al.* (*op. cit.*), in a systematic review of effectiveness of ways of supporting people with severe mental illness to gain employment, have evaluated the effectiveness of prevocational training and supported employment in helping people to gain work in competition.

Prevocational training involves the provision of sheltered workshops, skills training or transitional employment with a rehabilitation agency, as a method of providing a period of preparation before entering the labour market. Supported employment places individuals in jobs without preparation but with job support from a specialist in the workplace. The trials identified for review all took place in the United States, which limits generalisability, but the evidence from the review indicates that supported employment is more effective than prevocational training. Crowther *et al.* (*ibid.*: 207) conclude that:

> with the passing of the Disability Discrimination Act 1995, the UK government signalled its commitment to helping disabled people return to the workplace. People disabled by severe mental illness have particularly high unemployment rates ... the UK government should therefore encourage agencies concerned with vocational rehabilitation to develop and evaluate supported employment schemes similar to those in the United States.

This is something for mental health nurses to consider in the development of mental health services.

Health and physical working conditions

Our understanding of the effects of the physical work environment on health has changed over recent decades, partly in response to the changing nature of work itself. The decline in heavy industry has resulted in a diminution of adverse working conditions although the health legacy of mining and manufacturing industries still persists. The highlighting of physical risks of employment has been criticised (see Daykin 1999) for involving an overemphasis on the world of men's employment. Watterson (1999) explores how occupational diseases become defined and constructed as 'epidemics', thereby attracting attention. He notes the existence of 'silent' epidemics which 'have existed for many decades but have not been recognised by medical or governmental agencies for recording and compensation purposes' (*ibid.*: 109). One example is occupational bronchitis among miners, which was not recognised until the 1990s, when the numbers of miners had declined significantly. Mindful of such criticisms concerning an overemphasis on men's physical risks, occupational health concerns are now broader, encompassing psychosocial risks as well as physical, and attention to conditions of work in areas traditionally associated with women (Messing 1999). Nonetheless, as Vahter *et al.* (2002) demonstrate, there is still insufficient discussion regarding gender related differences in exposure to metals and the consequent health effects. Gender difference in exposure to nickel, for example, results in higher prevalence of nickel allergy and hand eczema in women than in men. Attracting attention to aspects of occupational health remains a political process.

In a global society, the 'old' epidemics of Western industrialised societies are becoming the 'new' epidemics of the developing nations. The concentration of economic power in multinational corporations has led to concern about globalisation of occupational hazards. The lack of regulatory systems in developing countries allows hazardous activities such as working with asbestos to be transferred. Whereas pneumoconiosis and asbestosis are diminishing in developed countries, they are increasing elsewhere (Johanning *et al.* 1994). Newer problems are being identified in the developed world, including occupational asthma and musculoskeletal disorders. One new area of interest in physical risks at work is that of the risk of passive smoking and the benefits of smoke free workplaces. Fichtenberg and Glantz (2002), in a systematic review of the effects of smoke free workplaces on smoking among employees, note that in the United States, passive smoking has been linked to the deaths of at least 53,000 non-smokers each year (Glantz and Parmley 1991). Smoke free workplaces reduce smoking. Through local ordinances requiring workplaces to be smoke free by 1998/99, 69 per cent of US workers employed indoors outside the home gained smoke free workplaces (Shopland *et al.* 2001, Fichtenberg and Glantz *op. cit.*). The results of the systematic review show that implementation of totally smoke free workplace policies encourages smokers to quit or reduce their consumption, reducing total cigarette consumption per employee by 29 per cent (Fichtenberg and Glantz *ibid.*). In addition, smoke free workplaces protect non-smokers from passive smoking.

Repetitive strain injury

As Canaan (1999) explains, the reported incidence of repetitive strain injury (RSI) in Britain has risen dramatically. She cites evidence from a Department of Employment workplace survey which found that musculoskeletal problems accounted for 550,000 lost working days in 1990, a figure which had doubled since 1983 (Khilji and Smithson 1994: 95). Rising incidence of this ill defined condition, involving symptoms of pain, pins and needles, muscle weakness, tenderness and loss of or limited movement, had been identified earlier in Japan and Australia, and now appear to be in decline in those countries due to attention to ergonomic principles (Canaan *op. cit.*: 146). The rising incidence of musculoskeletal problems can be linked to the greater use of keyboards by an increasingly wider range of workers and an increase in physical work demanding smaller and more repetitive tasks. Sewell and Wilkinson (1992) argue that just-in-time (JIT) production and total quality control (TQC) were two methods of organising work which ensured that just enough high quality goods were available to meet demand when necessary, leading to more intensive production patterns enabling greater profit for owners and managers, but subjecting labour to higher levels of surveillance, including control through membership of work teams. Psychosocial factors in the workplace may contribute to perceptions of physical health problems.

Macfarlane *et al.* (2000) have looked at the relative contribution of psychological factors, work related mechanical factors and work related psychosocial factors in the onset of forearm pain among a study population of 1953 persons in Altrincham, in the North of England, collecting baseline and followup data. The study participants were followed for two years through postal questionnaires. At two years followup 1260 participants completed the study questionnaire, of whom 8.3 per cent reported experiencing forearm pain. Onset of forearm pain was independently related to psychological factors, aspects of illness behaviour and somatic symptoms. Onset was also related to mechanical aspects of work (lifting or carrying weights and pushing and pulling weights) and to the level of satisfaction with support from supervisors and colleagues. Macfarlane and colleagues conclude that their study emphasises the multifactorial nature of forearm pain and argue that high levels of psychological distress and adverse work related psychosocial experiences as well as repetitive movements predict onset of forearm pain.

Coronary heart disease and work environment

Current interest in the relationship between psychosocial factors and the physical environment extends to a search for explanations for work related cardiac disease. As Marmot *et al.* (1999: 106) explain, coronary heart disease (CHD) arose first in higher socio-economic groups but then changed to show a pattern of higher rates of disease as the social hierarchy is descended. Furthermore mortality rates from CHD have declined more rapidly among higher than lower social groups, leading to widening health inequalities. When rates were higher amongst higher social classes, the assumption was that work stresses could be a contributing factor. As Marmot *et al.* (*ibid.*: 106) explain:

> The fact that CHD is now more common in lower socio-economic groups does not, by itself, refute the potential importance of work 'stress'. Research has moved on from the simplistic notion that high responsibility or dealing with multiple tasks represents work stress.

The increasing interest in the nature of the relationship between work and CHD is partly explained by the fact that although risk factors for CHD are now well known, the main risk factors — high blood pressure, plasma total cholesterol and smoking — account for no more than one third of the social gradient in cardiovascular disease. Marmot has argued strongly that explanations may lie in the nature of the social and economic organisation of societies. Evidence to support this comes from the Whitehall Studies of civil servants, which suggest workplace factors are significant, for reasons which have already been mentioned in this chapter: having a job brings economic resources; employment brings opportunities for personal growth and positive self identity; work brings social status and work brings demands on our time and energy. Changes in the nature of work in developed societies mean that fewer jobs are defined by physical demands, more by psychological and emotional demands, including the increasing number and range of jobs in the service sector which demand interpersonal skills. More jobs demand information processing skills and, as fewer jobs are secure and stable, there is an increase in part time and short term working and in job instability and unemployment (Marmot *et al. op. cit.*: 108).

Sokejima and Kagamimori (1998) have examined the extent to which working hours affect the risk of myocardial infarction through a case control study of men aged 30–69 in Japan, a country with comparatively low levels of morbidity and mortality from this condition, but with unusually long working hours (Uehata 1991). The case control study demonstrated a U-shaped association between mean monthly working hours and the risk of acute myocardial infarction. The risk of infarction was increased not only by unusually long working hours but also by shorter than average hours. The authors note that working hours may be shortened both by the presence of a premorbid condition, and by unemployment. Both these factors can increase the risk of infarction. A biological explanation for long working hours eliciting an acute myocardial infarction implicates changes in the activity of the autonomic nervous system:

> Work induced tension that increases sympathetic nerve activity increases blood pressure...in addition reduced activity of the parasympathetic nervous system increases the risk of coronary heart disease. It has been suggested that parasympathetic nerve activity is decreased by weak stressors that do not increase sympathetic nerve activity. Even if the stressors encountered while working are weak, coronary risk could be increased by attenuated vagal tone. (Sokejima and Kagamimori *op. cit.*: 778)

Explanations for work related psychosocial stress

There are two main models that attempt to explain the nature of work related psychosocial stress. These are the demand–control model and the effort–reward imbalance model. These models have been tested extensively over the past two decades, particularly through the Whitehall Studies of British civil servants. In the first Whitehall Study, dramatic differences in mortality by grade of employment could not be explained by known risk factors for coronary heart disease (Marmot *et al.* 1978). This finding led to a second longitudinal study — the Whitehall II Study of 10,308 male and female civil servants (Marmot *et al.* 1991).

The demand–control model

This model originates from Karasek's two dimensional model of work stress, where high level of psychological demands combined with low level of decision latitude combined to increase the risk of experiencing stress and subsequent physical illness (Karasek 1979). Karasek has also noted that learning may contribute to a worker's possibility of exerting control over the work situation (Karasek and Theorell 1990). The Whitehall Studies have examined characteristics of the demand–control model and found that the civil servants in the lower employment grades report lower levels of job control, less varied work and use of skills and a slower pace of work. Fewer of the lower grades reported satisfaction with their work situation (Marmot *et al.* 1991). Grade and psychosocial aspects of work were related to sickness absence. Jobs characterised by high work demands and low control predicted sickness absence (North *et al.* 1996, Marmot *et al.* 1999: 114). The detailed analysis of the results of these studies warrants further exploration (Marmot *et al. ibid.*); however the findings have had a significant impact on the direction of research in this area. An examination of the effects of work factors on coronary heart disease showed that 'both men and women with low control, either self-reported or independently assessed, had a higher risk of newly reported CHD during a mean follow-up period of five years' (*ibid.*: 115). Data from both the Whitehall II Study and a Swedish case control study (Theorell *et al.* 1998) indicate that a decrease in the amount of control over work over a long period of time was associated with an increased risk of myocardial infarction.

Separating out the effects of different factors which may be involved in the demand-control (or job strain) model is difficult. Relevant factors relating to the job are control over job, job monotony, range of skills used in work and pace of work. Relevant factors relating to the psychosocial aspects of the work environment are perceptions of support from colleagues and supervisors. Not all these factors are necessarily easy to measure and some crucial factors may be missing from the demand–control model. The role of self esteem and efficacy, for example, is more effectively explored in the effort–reward model.

The effort–reward model

This model maintains that the work role:

> is associated with recurrent options of contributing and performing, of being rewarded or esteemed, and of belonging to some significant group (work colleagues). Yet, these potentially beneficial effects are contingent on a basic prerequisite of exchange in social life, that is, reciprocity. (Marmot *et al.* 1999: 120)

The mechanisms of exchange are not necessarily within the control of specific work settings. The system of rewards — money, esteem and career opportunities — is influenced by labour market processes and societal values which in turn are affected by global changes. Changes in the labour market include job insecurity, fragmented careers and organisational downsizing which leads to redundancy. As a result there is an increasing issue around the effort–reward imbalance, that is a lack of reciprocity between the costs and gains of the work role. This, in itself, can lead to emotional distress and associated stress reactions through the autonomic nervous system (Brunner 1996).

Marmot *et al.* (*op. cit.*) identify six studies which have reported findings relevant to this model. The Whitehall II Study (Bosma *et al.* 1998) and a German blue collar (manual worker) study (Siegrist *et al.* 1990) found a two to sixfold elevated relative risk of CHD among those who reported effort–reward imbalance compared to those who did not report chronic work stress. High cost/low gain conditions were also linked to new psychiatric disorder in the Whitehall II Study and poor physical and psychological functioning (Stansfeld *et al.* 1998). Overall, the Whitehall II Study has found that both the demand–control and the effort–reward model were independently related to CHD outcomes, suggesting that both personal and environmental factors should be explored in examining the effects of work on health. The work of Marmot and colleagues has had a significant influence on the research agenda in relation to occupational health.

Organisational downsizing and employees' health

Kivimäki *et al.* (2000: 972) identify three mechanisms that link downsizing to health:

> firstly, alterations in characteristics of work, increasing perceived job insecurity and job demands and decreasing job control; secondly, adverse effects on social relationships — for example reduction in social support; and, thirdly, behaviour prejudicial to health — for example smoking and excessive alcohol consumption may become more prevalent.

From a prospective cohort study of 1110 public sector staff in Finland, Kivimäki *et al.* (*ibid.*) studied a cohort of 746 employees who remained in employment after downsizing. They found that major downsizing was associated with increased levels of physical work demands, increasing job insecurity, decreased levels of skill discretion and participation, lower levels of spouse support and a rise in prevalence of regular smoking. The effect was stronger on women than men and the effect on physical demands was stronger on those with low income than on those with high income. Sickness absence increased and most of the effect on sickness absence was attributable to changes in work characteristics. 'Increases in physical demands and job insecurity and reductions in job control, particularly in skill discretion and opportunities to participate in decision making' (*ibid.*: 975) were the most significant factors. The global prevalence of downsizing has led to an international research agenda about the health consequences (Ferrie *et al.* 2001, Kivimäki *et al.* 2001, Virtanen *et al.* 2002).

Brunner (*op. cit.*: 296) turns to John Ruskin (1977 [1851]) as a way of expressing concern about the effect of the occupational hierarchy on coronary risk:

> It may be proved, with much certainty, that God intends no man to live in this world without working; but it seems to me no less evident that He intends every man to be happy in his work. It is written, 'in the sweat of thy brow', but it was never written, 'in the breaking of thine heart'.

The occupational health of health professionals

Nursing literature records a wide range of occupational health risks for nurses. These include needlestick injuries (RCN 2002), latex allergies (Silverston 2001), back injuries, bullying and harassment by colleagues and harassment and assaults by members of the public (Blazys 2001). There is increasing attention being paid to the complexity of the health risks inherent in the demands of health care work and the culture and environment in which the work takes place. The demand–control (job strain) hypothesis has been tested with nurses through a longitudinal cohort study of 21,290 female registered nurses in the United States (Cheng *et al.* 2000). The study began in 1976. In 1996, 76.55 per cent of the 21,290 women followed up were working as nurses. As a longitudinal study, it allows the cumulative effects of job strain on health status to be considered. In contrast to the Whitehall Studies of civil servants in the United Kingdom, which found that high levels of job control were associated with high demands, in the nurses' study the demand and control scores were not correlated. The results suggested work patterns that included jobs characterised by high demands and low control and low demands and high levels of control. Work related social support was positively correlated with job control, but negatively correlated with job demand. Women with higher levels of job control, lower levels of job demands and higher levels of work related social support, reported significantly better health status:

> Women in the highest third of job demands and the lowest third of job control (reference group, 'high strain' job) had the worst health status, whereas those in the jobs with the highest control and lowest demands ('low strain' job) had the best health status. (*ibid.*: 1434–5)

Women with high demands, low control and low social support experienced the greatest decline in health status over time. Cheng *et al.* (*ibid.*) conclude that their findings suggest that strategies to reduce work related stress should include the redesign of jobs. Occupational health strategies that target individuals rather that the social environment of work will focus on the symptoms rather than cause of health hazards.

The peculiar nature of health care work and its associated strains are not confined to nurses. There is considerable concern about the health of doctors at a time of considerable change in the organisation of the health service (Williams *et al.* 1998). Thompson *et al.* (2001), in a Northern Ireland study of general practitioners' perceptions of the effects of their profession and training on their own health behaviour, confirmed earlier studies that embarrassment and unease with the role of patient contribute to self and mutual neglect. Doctors can be reluctant to admit to illness and a sense of conscience and of a high level of responsibility for patients, loyalty to GP partners, difficulties in relationships with partners, 'precarious sickness insurance arrangements, and poor locum availability may contribute to neglect of self and partners' (*ibid.*: 730). The sense of responsibility for others may be an important factor also in nurses' perceptions of high demands and low control over their work.

The prospect of an unhealthy workforce at a time when the health service workforce needs to expand has led the Department of Health to stress the importance of improving working conditions within the NHS. The 1999 campaign to *Improve Working Lives* (England) has led to the development of an 'Improving Working Lives Standard', published in October 2000. In 2000 The Royal College of Nursing conducted a survey of its members' wellbeing and working lives as part of its annual survey of members. The report of the *Working Well Survey* provides valuable information about nurses' occupational health risks. In terms of physical hazards, four per cent reported latex allergy, an increase from one per cent in 1999. Some 37 per cent reported that at some time in their careers they had received a needlestick injury from a needle which had been used on a patient, and seven per cent of all respondents had been injured at work in the previous 12 months (RCN 2002: 55).

A further significant health risk for nurses appeared to be bullying or harassment by a member of staff. One in six (17 per cent) reported that a member of staff had bullied them in the previous year. Some 34 per cent had been harassed or assaulted by a patient in the previous 12 months. The research used a psychological health measure, the CORE outcome measure. CORE (Clinical Outcomes in Routine Evaluation) is used to audit psychological therapy (Mellor-Clark *et al.* 2000) and is used in the RCN counselling service to evaluate the effectiveness of the service provided (McInnes 2002). The CORE outcome measure is a 34 item self report questionnaire which assesses psychosocial domains of subjective wellbeing. The RCN report notes that 'whether or not respondents were bullied or harassed in the last 12 months is the best predictor of CORE scores' (*ibid.*: 68). The proportion reporting bullying or harassment was higher (29 per cent) among minority ethnic groups. Some 41 per cent of nurses reported their immediate supervisor or manager as the main person responsible for the bullying or harassment. One third of those reporting problems reported they intended to leave the profession (*ibid.*).

Hockley (2002) has argued that the problem of interfemale violence among nurses in the workplace has been ignored. She sees use of terms such as horizontal violence or bullying as a reluctance to use unequivocal language to explore the problem. There is, however, evidence that nursing is beginning to address difficulties in the workplace (such as violence) that negatively affect the health and wellbeing of individual nurses.

The RCN survey also found that one in four nurses had taken sick leave in the previous three months and for a significant number (17 per cent of NHS hospital nurses) the absence was work related. Some 57 per cent of those with work related absence were not satisfied with their jobs. Nevertheless, half of respondents reported that their employer supported colleagues returning to work. Level of employer support correlated with degree of choice offered to nurses over their shift pattern (RCN *op. cit.*).

Control (or lack of it) over working hours was a significant feature of nurses' working lives. The RCN survey found that 43 per cent were not working the shift hours they would prefer.

Some 68 per cent of those on internal rotation would choose another shift system. Nurses working in GP practices and those on higher grades had more flexibility to self roster, but 56 per cent of nurses did not have this degree of choice. Staff who were dissatisfied with shift flexibility and control were more likely to have taken sick leave in the three months before the survey.

The overall importance of employer practice in providing a work environment which offered individual nurses an adequate degree of control over their work and appropriate levels of support was explored in the RCN survey through an overall measure of employees' views of their employer and two component factors, that is the extent to which nurses feel they are protected and supported by their employer ('protects') and the extent to which they feel valued ('values') (*op. cit.*: 63). The survey establishes a clear link between employment practice and nurses' wellbeing and identifies a range of attributes of a 'good' employer, including provision of a safe environment, protection and support, valuing staff, consulting employees and the quality of employee friendly services (*ibid.*: 69). The importance of many of these factors for nurses should, perhaps, be placed in the context of research which has identified the significance of low self esteem amongst nurses as a factor in their wellbeing. A Wales survey of 301 community mental health nurses, for example, has identified that although the group overall had average levels of self esteem a large group (40 per cent) were found to have low self esteem (Fothergill *et al.* 2000). Factors associated with low self esteem included alcohol consumption and being on the lower nursing grades. Length of experience was associated with high self esteem (*ibid.*). Hierarchy, status and feeling valued may remain problems for nurses.

In reporting on the RCN survey, *Nursing Standard* identified a range of good practices which illustrate the opportunities nurses have to contribute to improving their own and others' occupational health. Pearce (2002) reports on a 'zero tolerance sub-group' established by John Wells, a nurse working in a London hospital to help protect nurses from assaults by patients and relatives. The sub-group established a card system similar to the system used by football referees to warn individuals whose behaviour is unacceptable. Pearce also describes a self rostering system introduced in the intensive care unit at Doncaster and Bassetlaw Trust and illustrates the support provided through the RCN counselling service (Pearce *ibid*.: 12–15).

These few examples illustrate ways in which nurses can take more care and control of their own health in the workplace, and that of their colleagues, in accordance with the growing body of research findings that suggest that maintaining a balance between effort and reward and between work demands and decision latitude is important for a healthy workforce. The importance of social and managerial support at work may well be a key factor in feeling valued and protected by employers and by society in general. Feeling valued can, however, be particularly difficult for nurses as societal support for carers is at best ambivalent. Lloyd (1999) has argued that the wellbeing of unpaid as well as paid carers can be seen as an occupational health concern.

Occupational health nursing

The field of occupational health offers enormous scope to nurses willing and able and with a knowledge and understanding of workplace health and the skills to work with workplace communities as well as with individuals. Whitaker *et al.* (2002) surveyed occupational health teaching in pre-registration nursing programmes. Results of the study suggest that although occupational health is taught in over 80 per cent of diploma and degree courses, the subjects covered relate mainly to nurses' own health and safety. Broader discussions concerning how a client's health can be affected by work and how communities might be affected by employment opportunities were rarely addressed. Naumanen-Tuomela (2001a) has reviewed occupational health literature to assess the attributes of expertise and the occupational roles of occupational health nurses (OHNs). She found that OHNs held a wide range of roles, seeing themselves as expert, manager, leader, educator, advocate. Their work roles varied considerably but included work with individual clients, management responsibilities and cooperation with workplaces. In a further study of clients' views, Naumanen-Tuomela (2001b) found that clients had perceived a change in occupational health nurses' practice since the 1980s. OHNs' practice in the 1990s was perceived as being more client focussed, treating clients as equal partners and adopting a holistic, professional and empathetic approach to care. The increasing range of their work, however, meant that occupational health nurses had less time to spend with individual clients. Clients identified possible areas for development of practice for OHNs, including keeping their knowledge base up to date, learning to listen to clients and paying more attention to health and safety, health promotion, mental health and ergonomics. 'They could set up new groups for exhausted people and visit workplaces more often' (*ibid.*: 542) was a suggestion which reflects an awareness of the potential for occupational health nurses to make a significant contribution to workplace health.

Some authors explicitly promote an advocacy role for occupational health nurses. Such a role would be possible through making the most of their opportunities to liaise with employers to ensure that employees are supported in protecting their health. Dow-Clarke (2002), for example, argues that nurses have a role in assisting employees to achieve and maintain a work-life balance through advocacy for revised company policies. Hewitt and Tellier (1996) describe an occupational reproductive health nurse consultant role established in Wisconsin, thus illustrating the range of roles undertaken by nurses, and the breadth and depth of responsibility. The occupational reproductive health nurse consultant's primary responsibility was to provide advice and technical assistance about reproductive health, toxicology, industrial health and epidemiology to statewide agencies, organisations and industries as well as to individuals. Dyck and Roithmayer (2002) also identify a consultant role in occupational health, but with a different remit. They suggest that occupational effectiveness consultants should work with senior management to reduce the 'toxic cycle of harm' that can develop in work organisations. In this cycle, organisational stressors manifest themselves through employees' deteriorating health, productivity losses and escalating costs. Such a role could be seen as aligning occupational health with the interests of management. Johansson and Partanen (2002), on the other hand, advocate supporting trade unions in their efforts to promote health for workers and less privileged groups, arguing that capitalist globalisation means unions remain an important barricade in defence of workers' health and safety.

Bloor (2002) illustrates the role of unions in promoting occupational health and safety through a study of documents and oral history tapes drawn from the South Wales Miners' Library. Miners lived and worked with the tension between earnings and safety. In respect of roof falls, for example, each miner would have a section (a 'stall') of the workface to work:

> and he would be paid on piece rates, depending on the weight of coal he hewed. But each miner was also meant to ensure the safety of the roof, shoring it up with pit props supplied by the management, and of course the more time that was spent on shoring up, then the less time spent on winning coal. (*ibid.*: 95)

The miners and their families did not trust the coal owners to promote safety, a view which was justified according to reports of statements made by coalowners' representatives quoted by Bloor. Bloor reports Sir Evan Williams, chairman of the Monmouthshire and South Wales Coalowners Association in the 1930s as saying:

> Silicosis affects South Wales more than any other district in the country, and medical examination might prove many men to be suffering from silicosis who were not previously aware of it. And resultant claims for compensation would be inevitable. It is not thought to be in the interests of the trade to apply a medical examination to men at present in the employ of the owners. (quoted in Smith 1976, cited in Bloor *ibid.*: 96)

Unsurprisingly, the unions employed their own workmen inspectors who were responsible for examining the safety of the pits. Collective action to protect the health of the miners was grounded in class consciousness and a clear awareness of opposing interests between the workers and the coalowners. This opposition and lack of trust meant that for Dai Dan Evans, a union activist who became South Wales area general secretary for the Miners Federation of Great Britain, 1958–63, 'It was simply axiomatic that medical decisions on the level of compensation to be paid for workplace injuries would be dependent on the class (capitalist or proletariat) employing the clinician concerned' (Bloor *op. cit.*: 100). A doctor employed by the company would conclude a miner was fit to return to work. The doctor employed by the union would conclude he was not fit to return to work. Health professionals were perceived as partisan and the objectivity of medical evidence and medical judgment doubted.

The potential for the occupational health service to be perceived as supportive of specific interests raises many challenges for occupational health nurses. Winning the trust and confidence of the workers and management tests skills of empathy and negotiation and demands self knowledge and self confidence as well as an astute understanding of the workplace environment. The general theories referred to earlier provide different explanations of the forces that sustain workplace ill health.

Coronary heart disease, nursing and occupational health

A priority in tackling inequalities in health could be ameliorating the negative impact of employment conditions on coronary heart disease. A report from the National Heart Forum (NHF) advocates a unified approach across all agencies, aiming 'to create a culture in which a healthy lifestyle is a socially desirable choice, and an environment which facilitates such choices' (Sharp 1999: 146). Occupational health nursing is only one of a range of professional specialisms which can contribute to such a culture. Processes whereby work environments can inhibit rather than promote a healthy lifestyle are complex. There remains considerable debate about the relationships between physiological risk factors and psychosocial and behavioural factors such as high demands, low control, social support, coping strategies, negative emotions, exercise, smoking and diet. Investigating such relationships remains the focus for research. Recent work by Macleod *et al.* (2002), for example, has suggested that reliance on self report measures of symptoms of heart disease may have generated a spurious association between higher perceived stress and heart disease symptoms. Despite the need for caution, the significance of research concerning psychosocial factors conducted over a long period of time by Michael Marmot and colleagues continues to influence research and practice amongst a range of professions, including psychologists and nurses. Hemingway and Marmot (1999), in a systematic review of prospective cohort studies of the role of psychosocial factors in the aetiology and prognosis of coronary heart disease, identified, in healthy populations, an aetiological role for type A/hostility, depression and anxiety, psychosocial work characteristics, and social support.

There is particular interest in psychosocial factors and coronary heart disease on the part of those professional groups which may have a role in ameliorating stress. Psychologists have a particular interest and have developed interventions and approaches to investigating the impact of these interventions. Psycho-educational programmes appear to be successful in reducing key risk factors and heart disease. In a small study of 22 highly hostile men, for example, Gidron et al. (1999) found that a hostility reduction intervention programme reduced both hostility and diastolic blood pressure. Dusseldorf et al. (1999), in a meta-analysis of 37 studies of psycho-educational programmes, found significant positive effects on risk factors and on disease, although the programme had no effects on anxiety or depression. Steptoe et al. (1999) found that brief behavioural counselling by practice nurses led to improvements in healthy behaviour. This is a growing practice.

The possible importance of psychosocial factors alongside known risk factors such as diet, smoking, alcohol, hypertension and high levels of cholesterol, accords with nurses' self perceptions of the importance of their own holistic approach to care (Lukkarinen and Hentinen 1997, Wasling 1999). Nevertheless, developing independent roles in preventing primary and secondary heart disease is not necessarily easy for nurses. Occupational health nurses are not the only nurses with a key role to play in supporting a healthy engagement with employment. Practice nurses have a particularly important role in heart disease prevention and support. Moher et al. (2001) found that followup by nurses was as effective as followup by doctors in a trial to compare three methods of promoting secondary prevention of coronary heart disease (GP recall, nurse recall, audit notes with summary feedback to primary health care team). Wright *et al.* (2001), however, found that although nurses were effective in history taking, dietary advice and reassurance, they were less confident in discussing medication or patients' understandings of heart disease. (Nurses' confidence in discussing workplace stresses may also be limited.) Wiles (1997) has noted that for practice nurses to be able to provide high quality nurse led services, they need to be empowered through training, through opportunities to provide continuity of care, particularly through service integration across the primary and secondary care interface, and through raising of the status of practice nurses within the primary care team. Wright *et al.* (1999) found that planning services which address these issues supported practice nurses in playing a positive role. Change in services such as the withdrawal of cardiac liaison nurses after the ending of an integrated care project in Southampton (the Southampton Heart Integrated Project) had a negative effect on practice nurses' role in followup care. The most important factor in enabling practice nurses to expand their role was the support of doctors in the practice, thus confirming Wiles' view about the importance of practice nurses' status in primary health care teams.

An understanding of the importance of equal relationships and support for effective service provision within health care teams may help nurses understand the significance of workplace social factors in the aetiology of heart disease. There is no doubt that there are higher rates of disease amongst lower income groups. Baumann *et al.* (2002) report that the prevalence of hypertension is higher among lower income groups and there is greater morbidity. Wamala *et al.* (1999), in a case control study of Swedish women, found higher rates of coronary heart disease amongst those with lower levels of education and concluded that the increased risk was associated with lifestyle factors and with psychosocial stress. Poppius *et al.* (1999) looked at the relationship between sense of coherence and heart disease amongst Finnish middle aged working men. Sense of coherence appeared to have a salutogenic effect on white collar workers, but no consequent effect on the health of blue collar workers. However increasing personal perceptions of control and sense of coherence may not be the only protective ways of thinking about identity, life and work. Whiteman *et al.* (1997), in a cohort study, the Edinburgh Artery Study, found that 'submissiveness', a personality trait identified through a baseline personality scale (the Bedford-Foulds Personality Deviance Scale) may be protective against non-fatal myocardial infarction, particularly among women. These varied findings indicate the complexity of this subject area. For those in disadvantaged positions, the health consequences of demands, control, acceptance and resentment may be particularly complex to understand. Acceptance of one's position may reduce stress.

There is considerable evidence that appropriate services may not be accessible to target groups. The complexity of individual social and cultural influences has a significant effect on uptake of services and receptivity to health messages. Tod *et al.* (2001), in a qualitative study of use of health services by people with angina in the South Yorkshire coalfields, found delay, denial and self management were all factors that led to symptoms of heart disease remaining hidden from general practitioners, with consequent effects on appropriate referrals. The authors recommend community development strategies to improve access to primary care. Brown (1999) similarly identified ill health, preferences for other activities, money, lack of confidence and no one to accompany a person in the activity as significant barriers to exercise. Davison's work concerning the social and cultural reasons why people do not act on health promotion advice, and more recent research by Richards *et al.*, identify the complexity of factors which influence health behaviour in relation to heart disease. Davison (1994), in a study of the cultural construction of causation of heart disease in South Wales, found that there was keen interest in the long term effects of the physical, social and emotional environment of the coal mining valleys. The harshness of life had led to a culture of treats on special occasions — cream cakes, regular consumption of large amounts of alcohol, the 'take-away'. Davison notes that unhealthy behaviours can 'exist as elements of shared value systems that often have deep social meaning' (*ibid.*: 42). Davison identified two 'powerfully symbolic elements in the lay epidemiological system ... these images are both of people, and they appear to us as different sides of the same coin' (*ibid.*: 42). One is 'Uncle Norman' and the other is 'The Last Person':

> Uncle Norman is that happy character who figures in most people's social networks who has indulged in just about every risk behaviour known to medical science, yet has survived into a healthy old age. Uncle Norman smokes 40 cigarettes a day, eats a daily fried breakfast and has never taken exercise in his life. (*ibid.*: 42)

The Last Person, on the other hand, is the person who dies young and unexpectedly — the last person you would expect to have a heart attack.

The complexity of cultural responses to perceived risk and to symptoms of disease is further illustrated by Richards and colleagues in a qualitative study of socio-economic variations in responses to chest pain (Richards *et al.* 2002). Respondents from a deprived area in Glasgow had greater perceived vulnerability to heart disease than those from an affluent area but the greater feeling of vulnerability was not associated with reporting of more frequent consultation with a general practitioner. Those from the deprived area reported perceptions of self blame and fear that their lifestyle would be criticised when seeking help. They also reported normalising symptoms.

The difficulties in influencing individual behaviour often lead to calls for community based responses and interventions, particularly to address inequalities in health. The effectiveness of both individual and community programmes, however, remains unclear. O'Loughlin *et al.* (1999), for example, report on a four year community programme in a low income, inner city neighbourhood in Montreal. Followup at three years and at five years showed few community wide effects. Ebrahim and Davey Smith (1997), reporting on insignificant changes after interventions aimed at individuals, argue for fiscal and legislative interventions rather than community based or individual initiatives. Marshall (2000) supports this structural approach, arguing for a fiscal food policy that raises tax on sources of dietary saturated fat, thus reducing the likelihood that those living on low incomes will develop high risk dietary patterns. Tax revenue, it is suggested, could finance compensatory measures to raise income for those disadvantaged. These structural strategies may seem to be beyond the control of both patient and nurse, but they are policies suggested on the basis of ongoing and detailed analysis of the effects of inequalities on coronary heart disease. Understanding arguments for interventions at the level of society, community, workplace, and service provision, as well as at the level of individual professional practice and individual behavioural change, enables nurses to contribute to reducing inequalities in health and to extend and develop nursing practice.

10 Public health policy and practice

Margaret Miers

Introduction

The Labour government's policy emphasis on reducing inequalities in health was particularly clearly signalled by the Department of Health White Paper *Saving Lives: Our Healthier Nation* (DoH 1999c). This document makes clear that the government 'aims to attack the breeding ground of poor health — poverty and social exclusion'. The attack will involve an integrated approach 'to tackle the root causes of ill-health in places where people live'. The integrated approach will involve 'a three-way partnership' between individuals, government and communities. The route to better health is seen as through communities working in partnership through local organisations, 'delivering better information, better services and better community-wide programmes' (*ibid.*: 8). To illustrate how an integrated approach might work, the White Paper notes that:

> Reducing the impact of cancer and heart disease, for example, can be done only if we tackle smoking effectively. In turn, tackling smoking depends on relieving the conditions — social stress, unemployment, poor education, crime, vandalism — which lead far more people in disadvantaged communities to smoke than in other sections of the community. (*ibid.*: 10)

This emphasis on community wide involvement is matched throughout the White Paper with an emphasis on identifying health disadvantage. The strategies for health improvement advocated within the White Paper draw implicitly on the debates and research evidence discussed throughout this volume.

The theoretical support for the emphasis on the importance of integrated community action in improving health and diminishing inequalities lies particularly in the concept of 'social capital' (Putnam *et al.* 1993). Support also comes from Wilkinson's relative income hypothesis and Marmot's identification, through the Whitehall Studies of civil servants, of a gradient in health according to social position amongst those who are not poor. Marmot and Wilkinson (2001) continue to argue for the importance of psychosocial pathways in health inequalities. Contrary arguments include the view that it is absolute not relative poverty that leads to poor health, and the 'life course' view that it is individual material circumstances and biological capital rather than social capital that strongly influence health. Lynch *et al.* (2000) support a neomaterialist explanation, arguing that 'a combination of negative exposures and lack of resources held by individuals, along with systematic underinvestment across a wide range of human, physical, health and social infrastructure' (*ibid.*: 1202) provides the pathway to ill health.

Social capital

As explained in Chapter One, the concept of social capital has had a significant effect on public health research and practice. Putnam *et al.* (*op. cit.*) link the concept of social capital to that of 'civic society', a form of society characterised by civic participation, horizontal, not hierarchical networks, a sense of belonging, and values which emphasise solidarity and promote integrity. Interest in the concept of social capital has developed through exploring the relationship between economic growth and health gains. In his key article in 1992, Wilkinson noted that while it is known that as a nation becomes wealthier, its population becomes healthier, beyond a certain level of prosperity the gains in life expectancy are small and in some societies, the health gains are greater amongst the groups with the most wealth. Wilkinson (1992) argued that the overall health of the population, not just the health of the disadvantaged, is affected by income inequalities. Marmot and Wilkinson (*op. cit.*) document evidence for negative social effects of income inequality such as aggression, violence, loss of connectedness and reduced trust. In addition Wilkinson (2002) defends his relative income hypothesis through arguing for the importance of relations of subordination and dominance, drawing on Marmot's work relating to hierarchy and control in the work setting. Wilkinson recognises, however, that there may be problems in measuring variables such as domination and subordination. Data from the United States appear to support his views concerning the role of status, but European countries do not show the same relationships between relative income and health. He concludes that 'income may work as a better proxy for difference in social status in the United States than elsewhere. European differences in status ranking may be smaller and need more subtle markers' (*ibid.*: 978).

Support for the importance of social capital in affecting health and wellbeing has come from criminology. Rates of criminal behaviour appear to be linked to measures of social cohesion and feelings of safety. In criminal justice, restorative justice programmes in which the offender works in the community to support the social environment in which he or she has inflicted damage, are attempts to support the redevelopment of social cohesion. The Independent Inquiry into Inequalities in Health considered evidence relating to the health effects of fear of victimisation and recommended the development of policies to reduce the fear of crime and violence and to create a safe environment for people to live in (Acheson 1998: 55).

In the United Kingdom, health researchers are increasingly including measures of social capital in surveys that study the nation's health. The British Household Panel Study, for example, asks respondents about their neighbourhood and about community problems. An analysis of responses in terms of two measures — levels of social capital and levels of disorganisation — are used to analyse the data. An analysis of the relationship between these measures and psychiatric morbidity and physical health problems supports the relevance of the view that social environment affects health. People in the lowest categories of social capital had increased risk of psychiatric morbidity (McCulloch 2001). The Health Survey for England has also developed a set of questions to measure social capital. These relate to perceptions of the neighbourhood, its amenities and access to services, perceptions of trust and reciprocity, social support, participation and perception of problems such as vandalism. Answers to the questions concerning social capital also measure the degree of social exclusion (Bajekal and Purdon 2001). It is too early to say whether this major survey will support the importance of either social capital or social exclusion (or both) in understanding and explaining inequalities in health.

The importance of both building social capital and combating social exclusion is accepted in *Saving Lives: Our Healthier Nation* (DoH *op. cit.*). Although ongoing debate amongst researchers means it remains unclear whether it is relative income, psychosocial factors, individual income, material pathways or biological capital, which have the greatest effect on health, policy documents can recommend strategies that take account of all these factors. Hence *Saving Lives* recommends a range of factors to combat heart disease, including improving health in pregnancy, reducing smoking and tackling underlying factors through improving education, creating employment and improving employment conditions. Improving education, employment and the environment are all seen as part of the process of 'building social capital by increasing social cohesion and reducing street crime by regenerating neighbourhoods and communities' (*ibid.*: 81). There is also a strong emphasis on reducing social exclusion, particularly through action to reduce homelessness and protect the homeless and also through the expansion of Health Action Zones, which were first developed in 1998 in some of the most deprived parts of the country. An aim was to break down organisational barriers in order to develop an integrated approach to improving lives and reducing inequalities.

Further dimensions of social capital are addressed through the promotion of a healthy citizens programme that aims to ensure individuals have the knowledge and expertise necessary to take action on behalf of themselves and the community. Three developments are listed as 'healthy citizenship' projects (DoH *op. cit.*). They all emphasise enabling individuals to take responsibility for their own health and encourage involvement as citizens. NHS Direct provides accessible professional advice to any individual who telephones. The 'health skills' programme ensures health skills and knowledge will be developed throughout the population through schools, the Sure Start programme for parents, and investment in life saving equipment such as defibrillators in public places. The 'healthy citizens' initiative also acknowledges the importance of individual knowledge through an 'expert patient' programme intended to recognise the importance of patients' knowledge of chronic illness; the programme gives them more responsibility for managing their own disease.

The potential importance of feeling part of the community in which one lives is recognised through additional funding for measures intended to improve the physical environment of communities and measures to promote social networks. Sports facilities, community gardens and allotments, support for local shopping facilities and environmental strategies to encourage walking and cycling are all identified as important in promoting health. Successful strategies, however, depend on community participation. 'Real change can only come from the local community itself by harnessing the energy, skills and commitment of local people in setting clear objectives for change and forming new partnerships for action' (DoH *op. cit.*: 126).

Saving Lives also identifies strong roles for nurses, midwives and health visitors in the promotion of public health. Health visitors will be encouraged to develop a family centred public health role and to initiate and develop programmes to support health within communities based on local networks and expertise. School nurses will also develop their role as public health practitioners, providing support for healthy schools programmes, and guidance for sexual health and relationship difficulties. Midwives have opportunities to develop their role in serving vulnerable groups and providing preconception counselling for prospective parents. A subsequent government report has identified the need to develop public health capacity within the NHS through multidisciplinary training programmes (DoH 2001e). This report makes clear the importance of networking skills for nurses in public health, noting that 'the strategic programme for nursing and public health and the health visitor and school nurse initiative will support and extend the use of community development approaches among nurses, midwives and health visitors as a means of generating health improvement' (*ibid.*: 22). However additional skills also need to be developed apart from partnership working. Across the health workforce, there needs to be more awareness of public health needs, and the report argues that the need for a balance between clinical and population health perspectives should be acknowledged throughout primary care teams as well as in public health practice. It is recommended that an understanding of population needs be supported through the development of epidemiological skills and skills of analysis and critical appraisal of research evidence. Much of this development work is taking place through primary care trusts and through new university based postgraduate educational programmes in public health.

One of the underpinning disciplines which provides the evidence base and analytical tools for appraising evidence relating to population health is sociology. The examination of socio-economic differences in population health through understanding class and inequalities is central to the development of appropriate skills amongst health care professionals.

Evidence based public health strategies

It is helpful to consider the evidence base for the importance of social capital, material circumstances and individual life course in the aetiology of health inequalities alongside a review of different strategies adopted by nurses in community and public health nursing. The considerable challenges in this area are that arguments about causality are contested and that policies designed to effect change are expensive. It is widely agreed that health is related to income and to material factors. Muller (2002) however has argued that education is a more important variable than income, since income is dependent on education levels. Sturm and Gresenz (2002), in a study of common physical and mental health disorders, found no evidence to support the hypothesis that income inequality is a major risk factor. Evidence for the importance of material factors and the continued disadvantages associated with particular social classes comes from the fact that poverty tends to persist, both across an individual's lifetime, but also within communities, thus making it difficult to reduce geographical health inequalities quickly. Dorling *et al.* (2000), for example, have found that in central London, a measure of relative poverty and affluence of places made over 100 years ago remains as useful a predictor of current inequalities in mortality as the 1991 census. Not only does poverty persist in geographical communities but also in communities traditionally loyal to the Labour Party. Dorling *et al.* (*ibid.*) have identified the fact that the constituencies with a high proportion of Labour Party voters in the 1997 election were the constituencies with higher rates of premature mortality.

If poverty, or material aspects of life (malnutrition, cold, polluted air and water) act as the main population level determinants of poor health through having a direct effect on health, policy interventions should be to eliminate poverty and improve conditions. But as already explained, Marmot and Wilkinson (*op. cit.*) argue that the effect of low income on health is not direct. There is a psychosocial pathway created by the stress of relative deprivation, lack of social support and cohesion. They ask:

> If in the spirit of neo-materialism, you give every child access to a computer and every family a car, deal with air pollution, and provide a physically safe environment, is the problem solved? We believe not. The psychosocial effects of relative deprivation involving control over life, insecurity, anxiety, social isolation, socially hazardous environments, bullying and depression remain untouched. (*ibid.*: 1234)

Marmot and Wilkinson, however, make clear that their own emphasis on psychosocial pathways does not mean they would support policy initiatives based only on psychotherapeutic interventions. Structural issues such as absolute poverty must be tackled since it is the psychosocial factors that exacerbate the material disadvantage. This points to a multifaceted approach to reducing health inequalities, as favoured by the Labour government. Although the evidence for psychosocial pathways remains controversial, evidence for the effectiveness of interventions to improve material factors such as housing conditions also remains weak. Thomson *et al.* (2001), in a systematic review of intervention studies to improve housing, found very little research evidence to show that health gains result from investment in housing, perhaps because of the difficulties in conducting appropriate research. Raising absolute levels of income remains politically difficult without raising taxes and raising income may not be effective. Improving conditions throughout the life course, however, remains a main part of government strategy.

All public health practitioners face the possibility that their efforts to reduce inequalities in health may be ineffective. If psychosocial factors serve as a pathway for health damage, then community action to change the feelings of exclusion, deprivation, lack of control and lack of support may lead to health gain. If psychosocial factors do not matter, it would be more effective to provide additional income to the poor. If provision of income and material improvements do not have a direct effect on health, resources are wasted. Nurses have choices. They can work to alleviate poverty, as Hoskins describes in Chapter Eight. They can build community networks. They can provide new services, accessible in innovative ways. Varied nursing strategies are described below. As Davey Smith *et al.* (2001) make clear, when evidence is contested or deficient, that should not stop innovative policy and practice.

Tackling social exclusion

Health professionals did not wait for the 1997 election of a Labour government before making attempts to address social exclusion. Nottingham Community Health NHS Trust, for example, established a two year Strategies for Practice in Disadvantaged Areas (SPIDA) project in 1994. The project was based in an inner city primary health care team and tested an action research and team learning approach to enabling workers to develop empowering rather than victim blaming or state dependency strategies to alleviate the effects of poverty on children and their families. The primary care team developed a shared definition of poverty, which allowed them to place poverty in a wider context, and gave them a greater and more accurate insight into the lives of people in their community. Bond (1999: 13), writing about the evaluation of the action research project, noted that staff:

> were surprised to discover the extent of poverty amongst those on their list, particularly those in low paid work. It also came as a surprise to some staff to realize 'that people on benefits have so little money' and that some live in very cold homes. One person had realized that 'systems are not always conducive to sorting problems out even if

people go to the right place' and, for another, learning on the project had 'reinforced the link between poverty, asthma, eczema and the importance of breast feeding'.

One of the outcomes of the project was identified as growing collaboration between the primary health care team and other agencies. 'The practice manager joined a domestic violence steering group and a proposal emerged for a welfare rights worker to help health centre users to claim benefits' (*ibid.*: 13). Moore (1999) reports on a welfare rights scheme established in York, at the Clifton Health Centre. Health visitors, practice and district nurses and GPs are able to refer patients to a benefits advisor and appointments are made to see the advisor in a private room at the health centre through the practice receptionist. Staff perceive the advantages of this system as being able to overcome reservations about claiming benefits through linking benefits advice with health care. The holistic approach is welcomed by staff. Health visitor Hazel Stuteley's work on the Beacon Project in Cornwall has been recognised by awards and the attention of the Department of Health. As part of her role as health visitor Hazel organised residents' meetings and raised residents' concerns with councillors, police and teachers in order to stimulate action to reduce crime, improve housing, the environment and child safety. The importance of community ownership of development projects has also been demonstrated by a group of nurses engaged in community development in Bournemouth. Bournemouth University's Academic Centre for Health Improvement and Evidence of Effectiveness (ACHIEVE) has pooled the resources of researchers and practitioners to support local projects. One project which aims to improve women's health began with a public consultation exercise to identify priorities. These were access to cheap exercise facilities, access to cheap healthy food and access to information about healthy living. The Boscombe Health Action team developed an exercise class with crèche facilities and residents have now taken over the running of the project (Parish 2001).

Some of the most innovative public health and community work on the part of nurses has developed through Health Action Zones. In Cumbria, a former vascular nurse, Fiona Huntingdon, coordinates North Cumbria's dedicated stop smoking service with the support of ten home based, part time smoking advisers, trained in 'motivational interviewing' techniques. The aim is to take the service to the community rather than expect individuals to seek out professionals. Home visits are supported by hospital based group sessions. A midwife works with the team, taking special responsibility for helping pregnant smokers, and in 2000 the service was planning to extend into schools (Coleman 2000).

Luton's Health Action Zone has provided funds to expand and improve the cardiac rehabilitation service, thus enabling the appointment of a nurse as cardiac rehabilitation coordinator. The multiprofessional team includes a support worker for minority ethnic groups, a physiotherapist, an occupational therapist and an administrator. The team can refer clients to other services such as the smoking cessation service, and dietetic and clinical psychology services. This integrated approach facilitates 'a more seamless and patient-focused service through the phases of cardiac rehabilitation' (Dunkley 2000: 15). In Leeds, the 'action zone' concept extended to include dance, through DAZL (Dance Action Zone Leeds), a project which aims to improve young women's mental and physical wellbeing and access to exercise and health information through involving young people in dance. Dance is a performance and an energetic activity which can raise confidence and self esteem as well as physical strength. Fatchett (2000) reports additional positive outcomes including linking isolated young mothers and improved school attendance. 'Rock challenge' events are gaining national recognition and community nurses, nurse lecturers and researchers are providing varied levels of support through practice, education and research.

Awareness of nurses' role in addressing inequalities is not confined to inner city areas. Susan Davies adapted a 'Healthy Cities' programme to her work as a community project worker in Llanwrtyd Wells, a rural market town in Wales. Llanwrtyd Wells is part of the WHO Healthy Cities programme as it is a community with a higher proportion of people over 75 and 85 and a proportionately higher number of pensioners living alone than in the rest of Wales. It also has more households with three or more dependent children and a high percentage of people unemployed. The community profile indicates a high demand for health services. As a district nurse with a health promotion diploma, Susan Davies was well prepared for her secondment to the project. Her activities included linking with voluntary organisations and the local welfare officer to address transport difficulties and the failure to access appropriate benefits. She initiated discussions about agricultural accidents and, through funding from Child Safe Wales, she established a 'baby safe' course for parents. Since ending her secondments Susan Davies reported:

> My perspective on care has also changed. Since observing the effects that poverty, isolation and stress can have on people's health, the term holistic has taken on a new meaning. I no longer view clients' problems in clinical isolation, but in the context of their physical and social environment. (Susan Davies, quoted in Sadler 2002: 19)

Community profiling is an important part of the process of identifying priorities for action to address inequalities in health. Understanding the range of needs places individual needs in the context of the depth and complexity of disadvantage. Without an understanding of the community context, individualised care can reaffirm the relevance of Tudor Hart's inverse care law (Hart 1971).

Social inclusion

Nurses are also playing their part in reducing inequalities by developing services which include the socially excluded. Some of the most socially excluded are those in contact with the criminal justice system. The neglect of prisoners' health care needs has been widely recognised but health visitors are also extending their practice to include working with men on supervised attendance orders and young men and women known to the probation service. Black (2002) describes the award winning work of Audrey Anderson and Rebecca Jamieson in addressing sexual health problems and providing general health promotion advice, working with these groups in Gourock. Their work with these excluded groups was made possible by reducing the time spent visiting well children in their own homes.

Sadler (2001) reports on the work of Frederick Marais, appointed as the first TB/HIV clinical nurse specialist. He and his team work across health and social care boundaries to provide holistic care for clients who may be homeless or live in temporary accommodation and wish to keep their condition confidential. The nurses keep in touch with their vulnerable clients through community contacts and networks of professional and voluntary services. The nurses' listening skills, flexibility and public health knowledge support their practice with this excluded group. These are skills all nurses need in promoting an inclusive service, and in promoting public health.

Nurses developing services for homeless people have identified the considerable difficulties homeless people have using conventional services. The bureaucracy and hierarchy involved in many appointment systems, coupled with the regular change in personnel make it exceedingly difficult for services to respond to the needs of those without a residential address. Mental health problems and prejudice against drug users exacerbate difficulties homeless people face using health services. Voluntary sector workers have been perceived as providing more practical support and less judgmental care than health workers. However establishing separate services to meet the needs of this marginalised group may not be an appropriate approach. Gaze (1997) reports that a nurse run mobile clinic, a pilot project for homeless people in Manchester, was not considered a success. The nurses involved were not able to provide the specialist help needed to deal with drug, alcohol and mental health difficulties, nor were they able to prescribe medication. The nurses' view was that separate services further marginalise an excluded group. What is needed is to improve access to mainstream services. Walk in health centres may help improve use of mainstream services. An alternative approach is to provide one stop centres that incorporate health services alongside social services and facilities such as those for washing and a laundrette. One integrated service runs from the Harold Tomlin Day Centre, owned by Chester Aid to the Homeless. A medical team provides vaccination and immunisation programmes, advice on sexual health and minimising self harm. Dental and chiropody services and drugs workers are also available (Hampshire 2002).

The nursing press reports other more proactive approaches to social inclusion. Health visitors in Essex have taken part in a project to support people who struggle with literacy and numeracy skills. Such projects are supported by the Community Education Development Centre (www.cedc.org.uk) which aims to promote learning as a vehicle for social inclusion. Another particularly interesting project is a primary care scheme which involves participants sharing skills as part of the Rushney Green Time Bank, based at the local surgery. The scheme involves individuals identifying skills they have which they can use for the benefit of others in the community. 'Members deposit their time in their personal Time Bank account by giving practical help and support to another local member' (Beenstock 2001: 18). The scheme has 55 members and the main aim of the project is to recreate a sense of involvement in the community. Individuals with mental health difficulties and individuals living alone have particularly benefited from this method of increasing such involvement. The Time Bank is a practical approach to building social capital.

Tackling health inequalities: developing a sustainable approach

A sustainable approach to tackling health inequalities involves action in different arenas by different individuals with a shared understanding of public health priorities and of the nature of disadvantage. A sustainable level of activity to reduce health inequalities may develop from extensive and explicit individual awareness amongst health professionals. Few health professionals, on the basis of their own experience, can ever have doubted that social factors affect disease, but the extent and pervasiveness of the effects of such factors are now receiving closer attention from clinicians and researchers. Poor health outcomes through late presentation of symptoms are a common problem and one that is often seen as intractable due to the perceived inevitability of the social processes that support it. Late presentation with symptoms of colorectal cancer, for example, can be seen as an unwanted side effect of the reticence of the British in speaking sensibly about their bowel habits. But it is increasingly recognised that the reasons for late presentation may be linked to material inequality. Research into determinants of late presentation with glaucoma, for example, showed that late presenters were less likely to have access to a car and to be of lower occupational class than a comparison group with early glaucoma (Fraser *et al.* 2001). The researchers note that those with the least resources to cope with blindness are at higher risk of glaucomatous visual loss. Glaucoma, therefore, could be included in policies aimed at reducing inequalities in health.

The opportunities for nurses to help build a sustainable approach to addressing health inequalities are many. The government's targets for reducing health inequalities ensure that all professionals must think about the implications of their own practice and the service provided. The priorities for action are identified as:

- providing a sure foundation through a healthy pregnancy and early childhood
- improving opportunity for children and young people
- improving NHS primary care services
- tackling the major killers: coronary heart disease and cancer
- strengthening disadvantaged communities
- tackling the wider determinants of health inequalities through government policy (DoH 2001a).

The preferred strategies for action are to work with the community to raise awareness of barriers to health and to coordinate initiatives across schools, work, public, private and voluntary sectors. Nurses can raise awareness of health inequalities in their daily work with individual patients and clients, amongst work based teams, and in work with community groups as well as in management and strategic positions. A sustainable strategy to reduce health inequalities is one that is supported by individual nurses and by all professionals throughout the health service.

Is inequality inevitable? Sociology and scepticism

From the standpoint of the sociologist, a sustainable reduction in health inequalities may be viewed with scepticism. As Chapter One made clear, inequalities are a feature of all societies and social stratification is an integral part of social structures.

Different work is accorded different value, gaining different levels of status and resources, leading to differing levels of self esteem. Social interaction involves social support but also social dominance. Socio-economic groups, ranked on a social hierarchy remain and, in Britain, the legacy of capitalist class divisions still shapes regional, educational and employment boundaries in ways which can sustain or damage health. Sociology encourages nurses to review the effectiveness of individualised care within the context of social structures that limit the effectiveness of individual approaches to change. Drevdahl *et al.* (2001) recognise that the view that solutions to problems are constructed from the perspective of the individual is a feature of market principles in economics. They argue that this individual oriented, market led model of change is dominant in the United States. Population based interventions to distribute health more equitably are seen as attempts to rectify deficiencies in the market model of health care. Drevdahl and colleagues are sceptical, however, about the new popularity of the concept of social capital. They note that building social capital within deprived communities does not necessarily bring justice to those communities. They urge nurses to 'first create a climate of unacceptability for socio-economic differentials, including those in health' (*ibid.*: 28) and to recognise that building social capital is not necessarily congruent with social justice.

Thus, nurses, in synthesising knowledge and concepts from different disciplines, demonstrate the value of sceptical inquiry concerning the effects of social processes on health. Sociology's debates about inequality have moved on from debates about definitions of social class to debates about the importance of social capital, social exclusion and citizenship. Explanations for health inequalities remain many and varied. We still do not know if it is our levels of individual income or our sense of belonging and sense of personal control which have the greatest effect on health. Nurses, in their daily practice, explore and experience these issues and observe the process and injustices of health inequalities. This book aims to encourage nurses to broaden their knowledge and their scope of practice. More and more nurses are joining social scientists, policy makers and public health practitioners in finding ways to reduce the continuing effects of social class on inequalities in health.

References

Abbott P and Wallace C (1990) *An Introduction to Sociology: Feminist Perspectives.* Routledge, London.

Abbott S and Hobby L (1998) *An Evaluation of the Health and Advice Project: Its Impact On the Health of Those Using the Service.* The Health and Community Care Research Unit (HACCRU), University of Liverpool, Liverpool.

Abel-Smith B (1960) *A History of the Nursing Profession.* Heinemann, London.

Acheson D (1998) *Independent Inquiry into Inequalities in Health* (Chairman, Sir Donald Acheson), The Stationery Office, London.

Anthias F (2001) The concept of 'social division' and theorising social stratification: looking at ethnicity and class. *Sociology* 35(4): 835–54.

Baggott R (2000) *Public Health: Policy and Politics.* Macmillan (now Palgrave Macmillan), Basingstoke.

Bagguley P (1995) Middle class radicalism revisited. In Butler T and Savage M (eds) *Social Change and the Middle Classes.* UCL Press, London, pp. 293–309.

Baird K (1999) *Poverty and Teenage Pregnancy.* BSc dissertation, unpublished, Faculty of Health and Social Care, University of the West of England, Bristol.

Bajekal M and Purdon S (2001) *Social Capital and Social Exclusion: Development of a Condensed Module for the Health Survey for England.* National Centre for Social Research, London.

Baly M (1987) *A History of the Queen's Nursing Institute: 100 years 1887–1987.* Croom Helm, London.

Barclay J (1946) *Why Do Nurses? The Nursing Recruitment Problem, Its History, Terms and Solution etc.* Faber and Faber, London.

Barham P (1992) *Closing the Asylum: The Mental Patient In Modern Society.* Penguin, London.

Barker D J P (1992) *Fetal and Infant Origins of Adult Disease.* British Medical Journal Publishing Group, London.

Barker D J P (1995) Fetal origins of coronary heart disease. *British Medical Journal* 311: 171–4.

Bartley M (1994) Unemployment and health: understanding the relationship. *Journal of Epidemiology and Community Health* 48: 333–7.

Bartley M, Blane D and Davey Smith G (1998) Introduction: Beyond the Black Report. In Bartley M, Blane D and Davey Smith G (eds) *The Sociology of Health Inequalities.* Blackwell, Oxford, pp. 1–16.

Bartley M, Blane D and Montgomery S (1997). Socioeconomic determinants of health: health and the life course: why safety nets matter. *British Medical Journal* 314: 1194.

Bartley M, Ferrie J and Montgomery S M (1999) Living in a high-unemployment economy: understanding the health consequences. In Marmot M and Wilkinson R G (eds) *Social Determinants of Health*. Oxford University Press, Oxford, pp. 81–104.

Bartley M, Montgomery S, Cook D and Wadsworth M (1996) Health and work insecurity in young men. In Blane D, Brunner E and Wilkinson R (eds) *Health and Social Organisation*. Routledge, London, pp. 255–71.

Basaglia F (1981) Breaking the circuit of control. In Ingleby D (ed.) *Critical Psychiatry: The Politics of Mental Health*. Penguin Books, Harmondsworth, pp. 184–92.

Baumann L C, Chang M-W and Hoebeke R (2002) Clinical outcomes for low-income adults with hypertension and diabetes. *Nursing Research* 51(3): 191–8.

Beck U (1992) *Risk Society: Towards a New Modernity*. Sage, London.

Beenstock S (2001) Time share. *Nursing Standard* 15(46): 18–19.

Benzeval M, Dilnot A, Judge K and Taylor J (2000) Income and health over the lifecourse: evidence and policy implications. In Graham H (ed.) *Understanding Health Inequalities*. Open University Press, Buckingham, pp. 96–112.

Berney L, Blane D, Davey Smith G and Holland P (2000) Lifecourse influences on health in early old age. In Graham H (ed.) *Understanding Health Inequalities*. Open University Press, Buckingham, pp. 79–95.

Beynon H (1975) *Working for Ford*. E P Publishing, Wakefield.

Bhaskar R (1989) *A Philosophical Critique of the Contemporary Human Sciences*. Harvester Wheatsheaf, Hemel Hempstead.

Bissell G (2002) Follow up care and support offered to families post discharge from the neonatal unit. *Journal of Neonatal Nursing* 8(3): 76–82.

Black S (2002) Inclusion zone. *Nursing Standard* 16(16): 17.

Blackburn C and Graham H (1992) *Smoking Among Working Class Women – Information Pack*. Department of Applied Social Studies, University of Warwick.

Blane D (1999) The life course, the social gradient and health. In Marmot M and Wilkinson R G (eds) *The Social Determinants of Health*. Oxford University Press, Oxford, pp. 64–80.

Blane D, Bartley M and Davey Smith G (1998) Making sense of socio-economic health inequalities. In Field D and Taylor S (eds) *Sociological Perspectives on Health, Illness and Health Care*. Blackwell Science, Oxford, pp. 79–96.

Blane D, Brunner E and Wilkinson R (1996a) *Health and Social Organisation: Towards a Health Policy for the 21st Century*. Routledge, London.

Blane D, Brunner E and Wilkinson R (1996b) The evolution of public health policy: an anglocentric view of the last fifty years.

In Blane D, Brunner E and Wilkinson R (eds) *Health and Social Organisation: Towards a Health Policy for the 21st Century.* Routledge, London, pp. 1–17.

Blane D, White I and Morris J (1996c) Education, social circumstances and mortality. In Blane D, Brunner E and Wilkinson R (eds) *Health and Social Organisation: Towards a Health Policy for the 21st Century.* Routledge, London, pp. 171–87.

Blaxter M (1984) Equity and consultation rates in general practice. *British Medical Journal* 288: 1963–7.

Blaxter M (1987) Evidence on inequality in health from a national survey. *Lancet* ii: 30–3.

Blazys D (2001) Violence in the emergency department. *Journal of Emergency Nursing* 27(4): 352.

Bloor M (2002) No longer dying for a living: collective responses to injury risks in South Wales mining communities, 1900–1947. *Sociology* 36(1): 89–105.

Bond M (1999) Placing poverty on the agenda of a primary health care team: an evaluation of an action research project. *Health and Social Care in the Community* 7(1): 9–16.

Bosma H, Peter R, Siegrist J and Marmot M G (1998) Alternative job stress models and the risk of coronary heart disease. *American Journal of Public Health* 88: 68–74.

Bourdieu P (1977) *Outline of a Theory of Practice* (Nice R trans.). Cambridge University Press, Cambridge.

Bourdieu P (1986) *Distinction.* Routledge, London.

Bradley H (1999) *Gender and Power in the Workplace: Analysing the Impact of Economic Change.* Macmillan (now Palgrave Macmillan), London.

Brander N (2000) *Water Is Cool In Schools.* Enuresis Research and Information Centre, Bristol.

Brenner M H (1977) Health costs and benefits of economic policy. *International Journal of Health Services* 7: 4.

Brewster C, Mayne L and Tregaskis O (1997) Flexible working in Europe: a review of the evidence. *Management International Review*, Special Issue 1: 85–103.

Bridges J and Lynam J (1993) Informal carers: a Marxist analysis of social, political, and economic forces underpinning the role. *Advances in Nursing Science* 15(3): 33–48.

Brown J (1999) Barriers to physical activity in people at risk of coronary heart disease. *British Journal of Nursing* 8(8): 517–23.

Brown P (2000) The globalisation of positional competition? *Sociology* 34(4): 633–53.

Brunner E (1996) The social and biological basis of cardiovascular disease in office workers. In Blane D, Brunner E and Wilkinson R (eds) *Health and Social Organisation: Towards a Health Policy for the 21st century.* Routledge, London, pp. 272–99.

Bucquet D, Jarman B and White P (1985) Factors associated with home visiting in an Inner London general practice. *British Medical Journal* 290: 1480–3.

Burke L M and Harris D (2000) Education purchasers' views of nursing as an all graduate profession. *Nurse Education Today* 18(5): 368–79.

Busfield J (1986) *Managing Madness: Changing Ideas and Practice.* Unwin Hyman, London.

Byrne D (1999) *Social Exclusion.* Open University Press, Buckingham.

Callery P (1997) Paying to participate: financial, social and personal costs to parents of involvement in their children's care in hospital. *Journal of Advanced Nursing* 25: 746–52.

Canaan J E (1999) In the hand or in the head? Contextualising the debate about repetitive strain injury (RSI). In Daykin N and Doyal L (eds) *Health and Work: Critical Perspectives.* Macmillan (now Palgrave Macmillan), London, pp. 143–60.

Carmichael C L (1985) Inner-city Britain: a challenge for the dental profession. A review of dental and related deprivation in inner-city Newcastle upon Tyne. *British Dental Journal* 159(1): 24–7.

Carpenter M (1977) The new managerialism and professionalism in nursing. In Stacey M, Reid M, Health C and Dingwall R (eds) *Health and the Division of Labour.* Croom Helm, London, pp. 165–93.

Carpenter M (1985) *They Still Go Marching On … A Celebration of CoHSE's First 75 years.* Confederation of Health Service Employees, London.

Carstairs V (1981) Multiple deprivation and health state. *Community Medicine* 3: 4–13.

Carstairs V and Morris R (1989) Deprivation and mortality: an alternative to social class? *Community Medicine* 11: 210–19.

Carstairs V and Morris R (1991) *Deprivation and Health in Scotland.* Aberdeen University Press, Aberdeen.

Cartwright A and O'Brien M (1976) Social Class Variations in Health Care. In Stacey M (ed.) The Sociology of the NHS. *Sociological Review Monograph* 22, University of Keele, Keele, pp. 77–98.

Castles S and Kosack G (1973) *Immigrant Workers and Class Structure in Western Europe.* Oxford University Press for the Institute of Race Relations, Oxford.

Central Statistical Office (CSO) (1966) *Census 1961: Occupation Tables.* HMSO, London.

Chadwick E (1842) *Report on the Sanitary Condition of the Labouring Population of Great Britain.* Poor Law Commission, London.

Chapman H (1999) Some important limitations of competency-based education with respect to nurse education: an Australian perspective. *Nurse Education Today* 19: 129–35.

Cheng Y, Kawachi I, Coakley E H, Schwartz J and Colditz G (2000) Association between psychosocial work characteristics and health functioning in American women: prospective study. *British Medical Journal* 320: 1432–6.

Chiang T-L (1999) Economic transition and changing relation between income inequality and mortality in Taiwan: regression analysis. *British Medical Journal* 319: 1162–5.

Child Poverty Action Group (CPAG) (2001) *Poverty: The Facts.* Fourth edition. CPAG, London. www.cpag.org.uk/info/ Povertystats.htm

Chua W-F and Clegg S (1990) Professional closure: the case of British nursing. *Theory and Society* 19: 135–72.

Clement W and Myles J (1997) *Relations of Ruling: Class and Gender in Postindustrial Societies.* McGill-Queen's University Press, Montreal.

Clifford P (1986) Why I haven't joined the normies: some doubts about normalization. *South East Thames Rehabilitation Interest Group Newsletter*, London.

Cole T J, Bellizzi M C, Flegal K M and Dietz W H (2000) Establishing a standard definition for childhood overweight and obesity. *British Medical Journal* 320: 1240–3.

Coleman P (2000) The butt stops here. *Nursing Standard* 14(42): 19.

Colhoun H and Prescott-Clarke P (1996) *Health Survey for England 1994.* HMSO, London.

Connor J, Rodgers A and Priest P (1999) Randomised studies of income supplementation: a lost opportunity to assess health outcomes. *Journal of Epidemiology & Community Health* 53: 725–30.

Cornwallis E and O'Neil J (1998) Promoting health by tackling poverty. *The Hoolet* 18: 8–9.

Craig P and Greenslade M (1998). *First Findings from the Disability Follow-up to the Family Resources Survey.* Research summary no 5. Analytical Services Division Social Research Branch, DSS, HMSO, London.

Crombie D L (1984) Social class and health status: inequality or difference. *Journal of the Royal College of General Practitioners*, Occasional paper 25.

Crompton R (1989) Class theory and gender. *British Journal of Sociology* 40(4): 565–87.

Crompton R (1996) Gender and class analysis. In Lee D and Turner B (eds) *Conflicts About Class.* Longman, London.

Crompton R (1998) *Class and Stratification: An Introduction to Current Debates.* Second edition. Polity Press, Cambridge.

Crowther R E, Marshall M, Bond G R and Huxley P (2001) Helping people with severe mental illness to obtain work: systematic review. *British Medical Journal* 322: 204–8.

Culley L and Dyson S (eds) (2001) *Ethnicity and Nursing Practice.* Palgrave (now Palgrave Macmillan), Basingstoke.

Davey Smith G (1996) Income inequality and mortality: why are they related? *British Medical Journal* 312: 987–8.

Davey Smith G, Ebrahim S and Frankel S (2001) How policy informs the evidence: 'evidence based' thinking can lead to debased policy making. *British Medical Journal* 322: 184–5.

Davies C, Stilwell J, Wilson R, Carlisle C and Luker K (2000) Did Project 2000 nurse training change recruitment patterns or career expectations? *Nurse Education Today* 20: 408–17.

Davis I (2000) *Income Related Benefits: Estimate of Take Up In 1998/99.* Analytical Services Division, National Statistics, Department for Work and Pensions, The Stationery Office, London.

Davis K and Moore W E (1945) Some principles of stratification. *American Sociological Review* 10: 242–9.

Davison C (1994) Conflicts of interest. *Nursing Times* 90(13): 40–2.

Daykin N (1999) Introduction: Critical perspectives on health and work. In Daykin N and Doyal L (eds) *Health and Work: Critical Perspectives.* Macmillan (now Palgrave Macmillan), London, pp. 1–20.

DeBell D and Jackson P (2000) *School Nursing Within the Public Health Agenda: A Strategy for Practice.* Royal College of Nursing, London.

Department of Health (DoH) (1992) *The Health of the Nation: A Strategy for Health in England.* HMSO, London.

Department of Health (DoH) (1994) *The Allitt Inquiry. The Report of the Clothier Committee.* HMSO, London.

Department of Health (DoH) (1997) *A Bridge to the Future.* HMSO, London.

Department of Health (DoH) (1998a) *Strategy Launched to Modernise Mental Health Services,* DoH, Open Document (d400059763b) www.nds.coi.gov

Department of Health (DoH) (1998b) *Our Healthier Nation.* The Stationery Office, London.

Department of Health (DoH) (1999a) *Making a Difference: Strengthening the Nursing, Midwifery and Health Visiting Contribution to Health and Healthcare.* Department of Health, London.

Department of Health (DoH) (1999b) *National Service Framework for Mental Health.* Department of Health, London.

Department of Health (DoH) (1999c) *Saving Lives: Our Healthier Nation.* The Stationery Office, London.

Department of Health (DoH) (2000) *The NHS Plan.* The Stationery Office, London.

Department of Health (DoH) (2001a) *Tackling Health Inequalities: Consultation On a Plan for Delivery.* Department of Health, London.

Department of Health (DoH) (2001b) *Valuing People: A New Strategy for Learning Disability for the 21st Century.* Department of Health, London.

Department of Health (DoH) (2001c) *Working Together — Learning Together: A Framework for Lifelong Learning for the NHS.* Department of Health, London.

Department of Health (DoH) (2001d) *Reforming the Mental Health Act.* The Stationery Office, London.

Department of Health (DoH) (2001e) *The Report of the Chief Medical Officer's Project to Strengthen the Public Health Function.* Department of Health, London.

Department of Health (DoH) (2001f) *A Health Service of All the Talents: Developing the NHS Workforce.* Department of Health, London.

Department of Health (DoH) (2002a) *Tackling Health Inequalities: The Results of the Consultation Exercise.* Department of Health, London.

Department of Health (DoH) (2002b) *Health Inequalities National Targets On Infant Mortality and Life Expectancy: Technical Briefing.* Department of Health, London. www.doh.gov.uk/health inequalities/targetsupdatemar02.pdf (accessed 27/10/02).

Department of Health and Social Security (DHSS) (1968) *Report of the Committee on Local Authority and Allied Personal Social Services.* Cmnd 3703. (The Seebohm Report). HMSO, London.

Department of Health and Social Security (DHSS) (1980) *Inequalities In Health.* Report of a research working group chaired by Sir Douglas Black. DHSS, London.

Department of Social Security (DSS) (1989) *Income Related Benefits Take-Up in 1987–88.* HMSO, London.

Department of Work and Pensions (DWP) (2002) *Targeting Fraud.* www.targetingfraud.gov.uk

Devine F (1997) *Social Class in America and Britain.* Edinburgh University Press, Edinburgh.

Diez-Roux A V (1998) Bringing context back into epidemiology: variables and fallacies in multilevel analysis. *American Journal of Public Health* 88: 216–22.

Digby A (1985) Moral treatment in the York Retreat. In Bynum W F, Porter R and Shepherd M (eds) *The Anatomy of Madness, Vol 2.* Tavistock, London, pp. 52–72.

Dingwall R, Rafferty A M and Webster C (1988) *An Introduction to the Social History of Nursing.* Routledge, London.

Ditton J (1977) *Part-Time Crime: An Ethnography of Fiddling and Pilferage.* Macmillan (now Palgrave Macmillan), London.

Dorling D, Davey Smith G and Shaw M (2001) Analysis of trends in premature mortality by Labour voting in the 1997 general election. *British Medical Journal* 322: 1336–7.

Dorling D, Mitchell R, Shaw M, Orford S and Davey Smith G (2000) The ghosts of Christmas past: health effects of poverty in London in 1896 and 1991. *British Medical Journal* 321: 1547–51.

Douglas J W B (1967) *The Home and the School: A Study of Ability and Attainment in the Primary School.* Panther, St Albans.

Dow-Clarke R A (2002) Work-life balance in an industrial setting: focus on advocacy. *American Association of Occupational Health Nursing Journal* 50(2): 67–74.

Drevdahl D, Kneipp S M, Canales M K and Dorcy K S (2001) Reinvesting in social justice: a capital idea for public health nursing? *Advances in Nursing Science* 24(2): 19–31.

Drever F, Fisher K, Brown J and Clark J (2000) *Social Inequalities: 2000 Edition. A Report from the Office for National Statistics.* The Stationery Office, London.

Duckworth D (1877) *Sick Nursing, Essentially a Woman's Mission.* Longmans, Green & Co., London.

Duncombe M and Weller B (1971) *Paediatric Nursing.* Baillière Tindall, London.

Dunkley K (2000) Hitting the perfect beat. *Nursing Standard* 14(51): 15.

Dusseldorf E, van Eldern T, Maes S, Meulman J and Kraaij V (1999) A meta-analysis of psychoeducational programs for coronary heart disease patients. *Health Psychology* 18(5): 506–19.

Dyck D and Roithmayer T (2002) Organisational stressors and health. How occupational health nurses can help break the cycle. *American Association Occupational Health Nursing Journal* 50(5): 213–19.

Easterhouse Money Advice Centre (EHMAC) (2002) *Annual Report.* Easterhouse Money Advice Centre, Glasgow.

Ebrahim S and Davey Smith G (1997) Systematic review of randomised trials of multiple risk factor interventions for preventing coronary heart disease. *British Medical Journal* 314(7095): 1666–74.

Edwards R and Usher R (1994) Disciplining the subject: the power of competence. *Studies in the Education of Adults* 26(1): 1–14.

Ellaway A and Macintyre S (1998) Does housing tenure predict health in the UK because it exposes people to different levels of housing related hazards in the home or its surroundings? *Health and Place* 4: 141–50.

Engels F (1969 [1844]) *Condition of the Working Class in England.* Panther, London.

Engels F (1995 [1844]) In Davey B, Gray A and Seale C (eds) *Health and Disease: A Reader.* Second edition. Open University Press, Buckingham, pp. 125–34.

Ennals S (1990) Doctors and benefits. *British Medical Journal* 301: 1321–2.

Eriksson J G, Forsén T, Tuomilehto J, Osmond C and Barker D J P (2001) Early growth and coronary heart disease in later life: longitudinal study. *British Medical Journal* 322: 949–53.

Eyer J (1977) Prosperity as a cause of death. *International Journal of Health Services* 7(1): 125.

Ezzy D (1993) Unemployment and mental health: A critical review. *Social Science and Medicine* 30: 469–77.

Ezzy D (1997) Subjectivity and the labour process: conceptualising 'good work'. *Sociology* 31(3): 427–44.

Ezzy D (2001) A simulacrum of workplace community: individualism and engineered culture. *Sociology* 35(3): 631–50.

Faris R E L and Dunham H W (1967) *Mental Disorder in Urban Areas.* University of Chicago Press, Chicago.

Fatchett A (2000) DAZLing success. *Nursing Standard* 14(51): 14.

Featherstone M (1991) *Consumer Culture and Postmodernism.* Sage, London.

Ferrie J E, Martikainen P, Shipley M J, Marmot M G, Stansfeld S A and Davey Smith G (2001) Employment status and health after privatisation in white collar civil servants: prospective cohort study. *British Medical Journal* 322: 647–51.

Fichtenberg C M and Glantz S A (2002) Effect of smoke-free workplaces on smoking behaviour: systematic review. *British Medical Journal* 325: 188–91.

Fogelman K, Fox J and Power C (1987) Class and tenure mobility: do they explain the social inequalities in health among young adults in Britain? National Child Development Study Working Paper No. 21. Social Statistics Research Unit, City University, London.

Fothergill A, Edwards D, Hannigan B, Burnard P and Coyle D (2000) Self-esteem in community mental health nurses: findings from the all-Wales stress study. *Journal of Psychiatric and Mental Health Nursing* 7(4): 315–21.

Foucault M. (1971) *Madness and Civilization: A History In the Age of Reason.* Tavistock Publications, London.

Foucault M (1977) *Discipline and Punish: The Birth of the Prison.* Allen Lane, London.

Fox A J, Goldblatt P O and Jones D R (1985) Social class mortality differentials: artifact, selection or life circumstances? *Journal of Epidemiology and Community Health* 39: 1–8.

Fox N (1999) Postmodern reflection: deconstructing 'risk', 'health' and 'work'. In Daykin N and Doyal L (eds) *Health and Work: Critical Perspectives.* Macmillan (now Palgrave Macmillan), London, pp. 198–219.

Fraser S, Bunce C, Wormald R and Brunner E (2001) Deprivation and late presentation of glaucoma: case control study. *British Medical Journal* 322: 639–43.

Freidson E (1970) *Profession of Medicine: A Study in the Sociology of Applied Knowledge.* Dodd Mead, New York.

Freidson E (1994) *Professionalism Reborn.* Polity Press, Cambridge.

Gaze H (1997) Hitting the streets. *Nursing Times* 93(34): 36–7.

Giddens A (1997) *Sociology.* Third edition. Polity Press, Cambridge.

Gidron Y, Davidson K and Bata I (1999) The short-term effects of hostility-reduction intervention on male coronary heart disease patients. *Health Psychology* 18(4): 416–20.

Gillis A, MacLellan M and Perry A (1998) Competencies of liberal education in post-RN baccalaureate students: a longitudinal study. *Journal of Nursing Education* 37(9): 408–11.

Glantz S A and Parmley W W (1991) Passive smoking and heart disease: epidemiology, physiology and biology. *Circulation* 83: 1–12.

Godfrey J (1999) Empowerment through sexuality. In Wilkinson G and Miers M (eds) *Power and Nursing Practice*. Macmillan (now Palgrave Macmillan), Basingstoke, pp. 172–86.

Goffman E (1961) *Asylums: Essays on the Social Situation of Mental Patients and Other Inmates*. Pelican Books, Harmondsworth.

Goldblatt P (1990) Mortality and alternative social classifications. In Goldblatt P (ed.) *Longitudinal Study: Mortality and Social Organisation*. HMSO, London.

Goldthorpe J H (with C Llewellyn and C Payne) (1980) *Social Mobility and Class Structure in Modern Britain*. Second edition. Clarendon Press, Oxford.

Goldthorpe J H (1984) Women and class analysis: a reply to the replies. *Sociology* 18(4): 491–9.

Goldthorpe J H and Hope K (1974) *The Social Grading of Occupations: A New Approach and Scale*. Clarendon Press, Oxford.

Goldthorpe J H, Lockwood D, Bechoffer F and Platt J (1969) *The Affluent Worker in the Class Structure*. Cambridge University Press, London.

Goodman A, Johnson P and Webb S (1997) *Inequality in the UK*. Oxford University Press, Oxford.

Goulding J (1992) *The Costs of Visiting Children In hospital*. Action for Sick Children, London.

Graham H (1992) *Smoking Among Working Class Mothers: Final Report*. Department of Applied Social Studies. University of Warwick.

Graham H (ed.) (2000a) *Understanding Health Inequalities*. Open University Press, Buckingham.

Graham H (2000b) The challenge of health inequalities. In Graham H (ed.) *Understanding Health Inequalities*. Open University Press, Buckingham, pp. 3–21.

Griffiths S (1992) *Through Health Workers to Welfare Rights – A Report On the Health and Benefits Pilot in Goodinge and Finsbury Health Centres, Islington*. Camden and Islington Family Health Services Association, London.

Grundy L (2001) Pathways to fitness for practice: National Vocational Qualifications as a foundation of competence in nurse education. *Nurse Education Today* 21: 260–5.

Guardian, The (1997) *Underclass Now Knows Its Place in Revised Social Classification*. 15 December.

Gunnell D J, Davey Smith G, Frankel S et al. (1998) Childhood leg-length and adult mortality: follow-up of the Carnegie (Boyd-Orr) survey of diet and health in pre-war Britain. *Journal of Epidemiology and Community Health* 52: 142–52.

Gunnell D J, Frankel S, Nanchahal K, Braddon F and Davey Smith G (1996) Life-course exposure and later disease: a follow-up study based on a survey of family diet and health in pre-war Britain (1937–1939). *Public Health* 110: 85–94.

Hackman J R and Lawler E E (1971) Employee reactions to job characteristics. *Journal of Applied Psychology*. 55: 259–86.

Hadfield G and Skipworth M (1994) *Class: Where Do You Stand?* Bloomsbury Press, London.

Hallam J (1998) From angels to handmaidens: changing constructions of nursing's public image in post-war Britain. *Nursing Inquiry* 5: 32–42.

Halsey A H, Heath A and Ridge J (1980) *Origins and Destinations.* Clarendon Press, Oxford.

Hampshire M (2002) On the streets. *Nursing Standard* 16(31): 18–19.

Haralambos M and Holborn M (2000) *Sociology: Themes and Perspectives.* Fifth edition. Collins Educational, London.

Hart A and Lockey R (2002) Inequalities in health care provision: the relationship between contemporary policy and contemporary practice in maternity services in England. *Journal of Advanced Nursing* 37(5): 485–93.

Hart J Tudor (1971) The Inverse Care Law. *Lancet* i: 405–12.

Hattersley L (1999) Trends in life expectancy by social class: an update. *Health Statistics Quarterly* 2: 16–24.

Health Committee (1997) *Third Report. Health Services for Children and Young People In the Community: Home and School.* House of Commons Session 1996–1997, Minutes of evidence and appendices. The Stationery Office, London.

Heaney C A, Israel B A and House J S (1994) Chronic job insecurity among automobile workers: effects on job satisfaction and health. *Social Science and Medicine.* 38(10): 1431–7.

Heath A and Britten N (1984) Women's jobs do make a difference. *Sociology* 18(4): 475–90.

Heath A and Savage M (1995) Political alignments within the middle classes 1972–1989. In Butler T and Savage M (eds) *Social Change and the Middle Classes.* UCL Press, London, pp. 275–92.

Hemingway H and Marmot M (1999) Clinical review: evidence based cardiology: psychosocial factors in the aetiology and prognosis of coronary heart disease: systematic review of prospective cohort studies. *British Medical Journal* 318(7196): 1460–7.

Hewitt J B and Tellier L (1996) A description of an occupational reproductive health nurse consultant practice and women's occupational exposures during pregnancy. *Public Health Nursing* 13(5): 365–73.

Hicks C (1996) Nurse researcher: a study of a contradiction in terms? *Journal of Advanced Nursing* 24(2): 357–63.

Hicks C (1999) Incompatible skills and ideologies: the impediment of gender attributions on nursing research. *Journal of Advanced Nursing* 30(1): 129–39.

Higher Education Funding Council for England (HEFCE) (2001) *Research In Nursing and Allied Health Professions. Report of the Task Group 3 to HEFCE and the Department of Health.* HEFCE, Bristol.

Hirsch F (1977) *Social Limits to Growth.* Routledge and Kegan Paul, London.

Hobby L, Emanuel J and Abbott S (1998) *Citizens' Advice In Primary Care in England and Wales: A Review of Available Information.* The Health and Community Care Research Unit (HACCRU), University of Liverpool, Liverpool.

Hockley C (2002) The language used when reporting interfemale violence among nurses in the workplace. *Collegian: Journal of the Royal College of Nursing, Australia* 7(4): 24–9.

Hollingshead A and Redlich R C (1985) *Social Class and Mental Illness.* Wiley, New York.

Hoskins R (1999). It should be you. *Nursing Times* 95(33): 38–9.

Hoskins R (2001) Poverty and the health divide *Nursing Times* 97(25): 28–9.

Hoskins R and Carter D (2000) Welfare benefits screening and referral: a new direction for community nurses? *Health and Social Care in the Community* 8(6): 390–7.

Hoskins R and Smith L N (2002) Nurse led welfare benefits screening in a general practice located in a deprived area. *Public Health* 116: 214–20.

House J S, Landis K R and Umberton D (1988) Social relationships and health. *Science* 241: 540–5.

Howarth C, Kenway P, Palmer G and Street C (1998) *Monitoring Poverty and Social Exclusion: Labour's Inheritance.* Joseph Rowntree Foundation, York.

Hugman R (1991) *Power in Caring Professions.* Macmillan (now Palgrave Macmillan), Basingstoke.

Hunt S, McEwen J and McKenna S P (1985) Social inequalities in perceived health. *Effective Health Care* 2(4): 151–60.

Hutt J (2000) Young carers. In Muir J and Sidey A (eds) *Textbook of Children's Community Nursing.* Baillière Tindall, London, pp. 248–54.

Hutton W (1995) *The State We're In.* Jonathan Cape, London.

Illsley R (1986) Occupational class, selection and the production of inequalities in health. *Quarterly Journal of Social Affairs* 2(2): 151–65.

Jahoda M (1982) *Employment and Unemployment: A Social-Psychological Analysis.* Cambridge University Press, Cambridge.

Jarman B (1985) Giving advice about welfare benefits in general practice. *British Medical Journal* 290: 522–4.

Jarvis M J and Wardle J (1999) Social patterning of individual health behaviours: the case of cigarette smoking. In Marmot M and Wilkinson R (eds) *Social Determinants of Health.* Oxford University Press, Oxford, pp. 240–55.

Jenkins P M, Feldman B S and Stirrups D R (1984) The effect of social factors on referrals for orthodontic advice and treatment. *British Journal of Orthodontics* 11(1): 24–6.

Johanning E, Goldberg M and Kim R (1994) Asbestos hazard evaluation in South Korean textile production. *International Journal of Health Services* 24(1): 131–44.

Johansson M and Partanen T (2002) Role of trade unions in workplace health promotion. *International Journal of Health Services.* 32(1): 179–93.

Johnson T J (1972) *Professions and Power.* Macmillan (now Palgrave Macmillan), Basingstoke.

Jones K (1972) *A History of the Mental Health Services.* Routledge and Kegan Paul, London.

Judge K (1995) Income distribution and life expectancy: a critical appraisal. *British Medical Journal* 311: 1282–5.

Judge K and Paterson I (2001) *Poverty, Income Inequality and Health.* Treasury Working Paper 01/29. www.treasury.govt.nz/workingpapers/2001/twp01-29.pdf (accessed 23/8/02).

Kaplan G A, Pamuk E R, Lynch J W, Cohen R D and Balfour J L (1996) Inequality in income and mortality in the United States: analysis of mortality and potential pathways. *British Medical Journal* 312: 999–1003.

Karasek R A (1979) Job demands, job decision latitude and mental strain: implications for job design. *Administrative Science Quarterly* 24: 285–308.

Karasek R A and Theorell T (1990) *Healthy Work: Stress, Productivity, and the Reconstruction of Working Life.* Basic Books, New York.

Kawachi I, Kennedy B P, Lochner K and Protherow-Stith D (1997) Social capital, income inequality and mortality. *American Journal of Public Health* 87: 1491–8.

Kawachi I, Kennedy B P and Wilkinson R G (1999) *The Society and Population Reader: Income Inequality and Health.* The New Press, New York.

Kearns A, Hiscock R, Macintyre S and Ellaway A (2000) Beyond four walls: the psychosocial benefits of home: evidence from West Central Scotland. *Housing Studies* 3: 387–410.

Kehrer B and Wolin V (1979) Impact of income maintenance on low birthweight: evidence from the Gary experiment. *Journal of Human Resources* 14: 434–62.

Kennedy B P, Kawachi I and Protherow-Stith D (1996) Income distribution and mortality: cross sectional ecological study: the Robin Hood index in the United States. *British Medical Journal* 312: 1004–7.

Kennedy I (2001) *Learning From Bristol: The Report of the Public Inquiry Into Children's Heart Surgery at the Bristol Royal Infirmary 1984–1995.* CM 5207(1) The Stationery Office, London.

Kevles D J (1985) *In the Name of Eugenics.* University of California Press, Berkeley, CA.

Khilji N and Smithson S (1994) Repetitive strain injury in the UK: soft tissues and hard issues. *International Journal of Information Management* April: 95–108.

Kirby M (1999) *Stratification and Differentiation.* Macmillan (now Palgrave Macmillan), Basingstoke.

Kitson A L (2001) Does nurse education have a future? *Nurse Education Today* 21: 86–96.

Kivimäki M, Sutinen R, Elovainio M, Vahtera J, Räsänen K, Töyry S, Ferrie J E and Firth-Cozens J (2001) Sickness absence in hospital physicians: two year follow up study on determinants. *Occupational Environment Medicine* 58: 361–6.

Kivimäki M, Vahtera J, Pentti J and Ferrie J (2000) Factors underlying the effect of organisational downsizing on health of employees: longitudinal cohort study. *British Medical Journal* 320: 971–5.

Knight I (1984) *The Height and Weight of Adults in Britain.* OPCS/HMSO, London.

Kohn M and Schooler C (1973) Occupational experience and psychological functioning: an assessment of reciprocal effects. *American Sociological Review* 38: 97–118.

Koopman J S and Lynch J W (1999) Individual causal models and population systems models in epidemiology. *American Journal of Public Health* 88: 216–22.

Kuh D J L and Ben-Shlomo Y (1997) *Lifecourse Approach to Chronic Disease Epidemiology.* Oxford University Press, Oxford.

Langer T S and Michael S T (1963) *Life Stress and Mental Health.* Free Press, Glencoe.

Lash S and Urry J (1994) *Economies of Signs and Space.* Sage, London.

Lehman A F (1995) Vocational rehabilitation in schizophrenia. *Schizophrenia Bulletin* 21: 645–56.

Lelean S R and Clarke M (1990) Research resource development in the United Kingdom. *International Journal of Nursing Studies* 27(2): 123–38.

Lindsay B (2000) An atmosphere of recognition and respect? Sick children's nurses and 'medical men', 1880–1930. *International History of Nursing Journal* 6: 4–9.

Lloyd L (1999) The wellbeing of carers: an occupational health concern. In Daykin N and Doyal L (eds) *Health and Work: Critical Perspectives.* Macmillan (now Palgrave Macmillan), Basingstoke, pp. 54–70.

Logan W P D (1959) Occupational mortality. *Proceedings of the Royal Society of Medicine* 52: 463.

Lomax M (1921) *Experiences of an Asylum Doctor, with Suggestions for Asylum and Lunacy Reform.* George Allen and Unwin, London.

Long G, Macdonald S and Scott G (1996) *Child and Family Poverty In Scotland: The Facts.* Second edition. Save the Children Fund, London.

Lukkarinen H and Hentinen M (1997) Self-care agency and factors related to this agency among patients with coronary heart disease. *International Journal of Nursing Studies* 34(4): 295–304.

Lynch J W and Davey Smith G (2002) Commentary: income inequality and health: the end of the story? *International Journal of Epidemiology* 31: 549–51.

Lynch J W, Davey Smith G, Hillemeier M, Shaw M, Raghunathan T and Kaplan G (2001) Income inequality, the psycho-social environment and health: comparisons of wealthy nations. *Lancet* 358: 194–200.

Lynch J W, Davey Smith G, Kaplan G A and House J S (2000) Income inequality and mortality: importance to health of individual income, psychosocial environment, or material conditions. *British Medical Journal* 320: 1200–4.

Lynch P and Oelman B J (1981) Mortality from CHD in the British Army compared with the civil population. *British Medical Journal* 293: 504.

Macfarlane G J, Hunt I M and Silman A J (2000) Role of mechanical and psychosocial factors in the onset of forearm pain: prospective population based study. *British Medical Journal* 321: 676–9.

MacGuire J M (1969) *Threshold to Nursing: A Review of the Literature On Recruitment to and Withdrawal from Nurse Training Programmes In the United Kingdom.* Bell, London.

Macintyre S (1997) The Black Report and beyond: what are the issues? *Social Science and Medicine* 44(6): 723–45.

Macintyre S, Ellaway A, Der G, Ford G and Hunt K (1998) Are housing tenure and car access simply markers of income or self esteem? A Scottish study. *Journal of Epidemiology and Community Health* 52: 657–64.

Macintyre S, Hiscock R, Kearns A and Ellaway A (2000) Housing tenure and health inequalities: a three dimensional perspective on people, homes and neighbourhoods. In Graham H (ed.) *Understanding Health Inequalities.* Open University Press, Buckingham, pp. 129–42.

Macleod J, Davey Smith G, Heslop P, Metcalfe C, Carroll D and Hart C (2002) Psychological stress and cardiovascular disease: empirical demonstration of bias in a prospective observational study of Scottish men. *British Medical Journal* 324: 1247–51.

Maggs C J (1983) *The Origins of General Nursing.* Croom Helm, London.

Marmot M G (1999) Introduction. In Marmot M and Wilkinson R G (eds) *Social Determinants of Health.* Oxford University Press, Oxford, pp. 1–16.

Marmot M G and Davey Smith G (1989) Why are the Japanese living longer? *British Medical Journal* 299: 1547–51.

Marmot M G and Shipley M J (1996) Do socio-economic differences persist after retirement? Twenty-five year follow up of civil servants from the first Whitehall Study. *British Medical Journal* 313: 1177–80.

Marmot M G and Syme S L (1976) Acculturation and coronary heart disease in Japanese Americans. *American Journal of Epidemiology* 104: 225–47.

Marmot M G and Wadsworth M E J (1997) *Fetal and Early Childhood Environment: Long Term Implications.* Churchill Livingstone, Edinburgh.

Marmot M G and Wilkinson R G (eds) (1999) *Social Determinants of Health*. Oxford University Press, Oxford.

Marmot M G and Wilkinson R G (2001) Psychosocial and material pathways in the relation between income and health: a response to Lynch *et al*. *British Medical Journal* 322: 1233–5.

Marmot M G, Bosma H, Hemingway H, Brunner E and Stansfield S (1997) Contributions of job control and other risk factors to social variations in coronary heart disease incidence. *Lancet* 350: 235–9.

Marmot M G, Davey Smith G, Stansfield S, Patel C, North F and Head J (1991) Health inequalities among British civil servants: the Whitehall II Study. *Lancet* 337: 1387–93.

Marmot M G, Rose G, Shipley M and Hamilton P J S (1978) Employment grade and coronary heart disease in British civil servants. *Journal of Epidemiology and Community Health* 32: 244–9.

Marmot M G, Shipley M J and Rose G (1984) Inequalities in death – specific explanations of a general pattern? *Lancet* i: 1003–6.

Marmot M G, Siegrist J, Theorell T and Feeney A (1999) Health and the psychosocial environment at work. In Marmot M and Wilkinson R G (eds) *Social Determinants of Health*. Oxford University Press, Oxford, pp. 105–31.

Marsh G N and Channing D M (1986) Deprivation and health in one general practice. *British Medical Journal* 292: 1173–6.

Marshall T (2000) Exploring a fiscal food policy: the case of diet and ischaemic heart disease. *British Medical Journal* 320: 301–5.

Marshall T H (1950) *Citizenship and Social Class and Other Essays*, Cambridge: Cambridge University Press.

Marshall T H (1963) Citizenship and social class. In Marshall T H (ed.) *Sociology At the Crossroads*. Heinemann, London.

Martin J (1998) A new definition for the household reference person. *Survey Methodology Bulletin* 43: 1–8.

Marx K and Engels F (1967) *The Communist Manifesto*. Penguin, Harmondsworth.

Marx K and Engels F (1995) Karl Marx and Friedrich Engels on Class. In Joyce P (ed.) *Class*. Oxford University Press, Oxford, pp. 21–30.

Mayall B (1994) *Negotiating Health: Primary School Children at Home and School*. Cassell, London.

McCulloch A (2001) Social environments and health: cross sectional national survey. *British Medical Journal* 323: 208–9.

McInnes B (2002) Vicious cycle. *Nursing Standard* 16(27): 14–15.

McKenna H (2000) Personal communication.

McKibbin R (1990) *The Ideologies of Class*. Oxford University Press, Oxford.

McLoone P and Boddy F A (1994) Deprivation and mortality in Scotland, 1981 and 1991. *British Medical Journal* 309: 1465–70.

Mellor-Clark J, Barkham M, Connell J and Evans C (2000) Practice based evidence and need for a standardised evaluation system: informing the design of the CORE System. *European Journal of Psychotherapy, Counselling and Health* 2(3): 357–74.

Meltzer H, Gill B, Petticrew M and Hinds K (1995) *Economic Activity and Social Functioning of Adults with Psychiatric Disorders*. HMSO, London.

Messing K (1999) Tracking the invisible: scientific indicators of the health hazards of women's work. In Daykin N and Doyal L (eds) *Health and Work: Critical Perspectives*. Macmillan (now Palgrave Macmillan), Basingstoke, pp. 127–42.

Middleton J, Spearey H, Maunder B, Vanes J, Little V, Norman A, Bentley D, Lucas G and Bone B (1993) Citizen's advice in general practice (letter). *British Medical Journal* 307(6902): 504.

Middleton S (1987) Streaming and the politics of female sexuality: case studies in the schooling of girls. In Weiner G and Arnot M (eds) *Gender Under Scrutiny: New Inquiries In Education*. Unwin Hyman, London, pp. 102–17.

Miers M (1999) Nurses in the labour market: exploring and explaining nurses' work. In Wilkinson G and Miers M (eds) *Power and Nursing Practice*. Macmillan (now Palgrave Macmillan), Basingstoke, pp. 83–96.

Miers M (2000) *Gender Issues and Nursing Practice*. Macmillan (now Palgrave Macmillan), Basingstoke.

Miers M (2002a) Developing an understanding of gender sensitive care: exploring concepts and knowledge. *Journal of Advanced Nursing* 40(1): 69–77.

Miers M (2002b) Nurse education in higher education: understanding cultural barriers to progress. *Nurse Education Today* 22: 212–19.

Milligan F (1998) Defining and assessing competence: the distraction of outcomes and the importance of the educational process. *Nurse Education Today* 18: 273–80.

MIND (1961) *Report of the Annual Conference of the National Association for Mental Health*. MIND, London, at pp. 4–10.

Ministry of Agriculture, Fisheries and Food (MAFF) (1977) *Household Food Consumption and Expenditure 1976: Annual Report of the National Food Survey Committee*. HMSO, London.

Ministry of Agriculture, Fisheries and Food (MAFF) (1986) *Household Food Consumption and Expenditure 1984: Annual Report of the National Food Survey Committee*. HMSO, London.

Ministry of Health (1959) *The Welfare of Children in Hospital: A Report of the Committee*. HMSO, London.

Mitchell D (2000) Nursing and social policy in the 1930s: a discussion of mental deficiency nursing. *International History of Nursing Journal* 6: 56–61.

Moher M, Yudkin P, Wright L, Turner R, Fuller A, Schofield T and Mant D (2001) Cluster randomised controlled trail to compare three methods of promoting secondary prevention of coronary heart disease in primary care. *British Medical Journal* 322: 1338–42.

Montgomery S M, Cook D G, Bartley M J and Wadsworth M E J (1999) Unemployment in young men pre-dates symptoms of depression and anxiety resulting in medical consultation. *International Journal of Epidemiology* 28: 95–100.

Moore A (1999) Benefits check-up. *Nursing Standard* 13(41): 17.

Morris J K, Cook D G and Shaper A G (1994) Loss of employment and mortality. *British Medical Journal* 308: 1135–9.

Moser K A, Fox A J and Jones D R (1984) Unemployment and mortality in the OPCS Longitudinal Study. *Lancet* ii: 1324–8.

Muir J and Sidey A (2000) *Textbook of Community Children's Nursing*. Baillière Tindall/RCN, London.

Muller A (2002) Education, income inequality, and mortality: a multiple regression analysis. *British Medical Journal* 324: 23–5.

Multiple Risk Factor Intervention Trial Research Group (1982) The Multiple Risk Factor Intervention Trial: risk factor changes and mortality results. *Journal of the American Medical Association* 248: 1465–76.

Murphy R (1984) The structure of closure: A critique and development of the theories of Weber, Collins and Parkin. *British Journal of Sociology* 35: 547–67.

Murray C A (1990) *The Emerging British Underclass*. Institute of Economic Analysis Health and Welfare Unit, London.

Murray C A (1994) *Underclass: The Crisis Deepens*. Institute of Economic Analysis Health and Welfare Unit, London.

Naidoo J and Wills J (1998) *Practising Health Promotion: Dilemmas and Challenges*. Baillière Tindall, London.

Naumanen-Tuomela P (2001a) Concept analysis of expertise of occupational health nurses applying Rodgers's evolutionary model. *International Journal of Nursing Practice* 7(4): 257–65.

Naumanen-Tuomela P (2001b) Finnish occupational health nurses' work and expertise: the clients' perspective. *Journal of Advanced Nursing* 34(4): 538–44.

Nettleton S and Burrows R (1998) Mortgage debt, insecure home ownership and health: an exploratory analysis. *Sociology of Health and Illness* 20(5): 731–53.

Newell P (1991) *The UN Convention and Children's Rights in the UK*. NCB, London.

Newman T and Roberts H (2001) Reducing inequalities in child health. *Professional Care of Mother and Child* 11(4): 90–1.

Nolan P (1991) Looking at the first 100 years. *Senior Nurse* 11: 22–5.

Nolan P (1995) Mental health nursing: origins and developments. In Baly M (ed.) *Nursing and Social Change*. Third edition. Routledge, London, pp. 250–63.

Nordenmark M and Strandh M (1999) Towards a sociological understanding of mental well-being among the unemployed: the role of economic and psychosocial factors. *Sociology* 33(3): 577–97.

North Derbyshire RDA Project 317/95/0010 (1997) *Welfare Rights In Primary Care (Shirebrook and Bolsover Practices,*

Derbyshire): First Annual Report 14 April 1996–31 March 1997. Derbyshire County Council Welfare Rights Service, Derby.

North F M, Syme S L, Feeney A, Shipley M and Marmot M G (1996) Psychosocial work environment and sickness absence among British civil servants: The Whitehall II Study. *American Journal of Public Health* 86: 332–40.

North Tyneside Citizens' Advice Bureau (1997) *North Tyneside Citizens' Advice Bureau Health Centre Service Annual Report 1996–1997.* Newcastle upon Tyne, North Tyneside Citizens' Advice Bureau.

Nursing Times (1999) RCN reviews nurses' role in benefit uptake. *Nursing Times* 95(28): 12–13.

Nylén L, Voss M and Floderus B (2001) Mortality among women and men relative to unemployment, part-time work, overtime work and extra work: a study based on data from the Swedish twin registry. *Occupational and Environmental Medicine.* 58(1): 52–7.

Oakley A (1974) *The Sociology of Housework.* Martin Robertson, London.

O'Connor J (1973) *The Fiscal Crisis of The State.* Martin Press, New York.

Office for National Statistics (2001a) *The National Statistics Socio-Economic Classification.* ONS, London.

Office for National Statistics (ONS) (2001b) *National Statistics Annual Report 2000–2001.* ONS, London.

Office for National Statistics (ONS) (2001c) *Economic Trends. Taxes and Benefits: The Effects on Household Income.* ONS, London.

Office for Population Censuses and Surveys (OPCS) (1978) *Occupational Mortality, Decennial Supplement, 1970–72, England and Wales.* HMSO, London.

Oliver M (1990) *The Politics of Disablement.* Macmillan (now Palgrave Macmillan), London.

O'Loughlin J L, Paradis G, Gray-Donald K and Renaud L (1999) The impact of a community-based heart disease prevention program in a low-income, inner city neighbourhood. *American Journal of Public Health* 89(12): 1819–26.

Oppenheim C and Harker L (1996) *Poverty: The Facts.* Child Poverty Action Group, London.

Osler M, Prescott E, Gronbaek M, Christensen U, Due P and Engholm G (2002) Income inequality, individual income, and mortality in Danish adults: analysis of pooled data from two cohort studies. *British Medical Journal* 324: 13–16.

Pakulski J and Waters M (1996) *The Death of Class.* Sage, London.

Pantry S (1995) *Occupational Health.* Chapman Hall, London.

Paris J A G and Player D (1993) Citizen's advice in general practice. *British Medical Journal* 306: 1518–20.

Parish C (2001) You've got the power. *Nursing Standard* 15(29): 18–19.

Parkin F (1979) *Marxism and Class Theory: A Bourgeois Critique.* Tavistock, London.

Parsons T (1951) *The Social System.* The Free Press, New York.

Pearce L (2002) Are you working well? *Nursing Standard* 16(27): 12–15.

Pelling M (1978) *Cholera, Fever and English Medicine 1825–65.* Oxford University Press, Oxford.

Pendleton D A and Bochner S (1980) The communication of medical information in general practice consultations as a function of patients' social class. *Social Science and Medicine* 14: 669–73.

Philhammar Andersson E (1999) From vocational training to academic education: the situation of the schools of nursing in Sweden. *Journal of Nursing Education* 38(1): 33–8.

Phillimore P, Beattie A and Townsend P (1994) Widening inequality of health in northern England 1981–1991. *British Medical Journal* 308: 1125–8.

Popay J, Williams G, Thomas C and Gatrell A (1998) Theorising inequalities in health: the place of lay knowledge. In Bartley M, Blane D and Davey Smith G (eds) *The Sociology of Health Inequalities.* Blackwell, Oxford, pp. 59–83.

Poppius E, Tenkanen L, Kalimo R and Heinsalmi P (1999) The sense of coherence, occupation and risk of coronary heart disease in the Helsinki Heart Study. *Social Science and Medicine* 49(1): 109–20.

Porter R (1992) Foucault's great confinement. In Stills A and Velody I (eds) *Rewriting the History of Madness.* Routledge, London, pp. 119–26.

Porter S (1998) *Social Theory and Nursing Practice.* Palgrave (now Palgrave Macmillan), Basingstoke.

Power C, Manor O and Fox J (1991) *Health and Class: The Early Years.* Chapman and Hall, London.

Power C, Matthews S and Manor O (1996) Inequalities in self rated health in the 1958 birth cohort: lifetime social circumstances or social mobility? *British Medical Journal* 313: 449–53.

Prandy K (1990) The revised Cambridge scale of occupations. *Sociology* 24: 629–55.

Prescott-Clarke P and Primatesta P (1998) *Health Survey for England 1996.* The Stationery Office, London.

Prior L (1991) Community versus hospital care: the crisis in psychiatric provision. *Social Science and Medicine* 32(4): 483–9.

Putnam R D, Leonardi R and Nanetti R Y (1993) *Making Democracy Work: Civic Traditions in Modern Italy.* Princeton University Press, Princeton, NJ.

Pyramid Trust www.nptrust.orguk/evid.html (accessed 30/09/02).

Quick A and Wilkinson R G (1991) *Income and Health.* Socialist Health Association, London.

Rae M (2000) The past, present and future: Stanley Moore Memorial Lecture. Paper presented at the Community Psychiatric

Nursing Association Annual Conference, 29 March, University of York, York.

Rafferty A M (1995) The anomaly of autonomy: space and status in early nursing reform. *International History of Nursing Journal* 1: 43–56.

Rafferty A M (1996) *The Politics of Nursing Knowledge.* Routledge, London.

Ramon S (1985) *Psychiatry in Britain: Meaning and Policy.* Croom Helm, Beckenham.

Read J and Baker S (1996) *Not Just Sticks and Stones: A Survey of the Stigma, Taboos and Discrimination Experienced by People with Mental Health Problems.* MIND, London.

Reading R, Langford I, Haynes R, Lovett A (1999) Accidents to preschool children: comparing family and neighbourhood risk factors. *Social Science and Medicine* 48(3): 3321–30.

Reay D, Davies J, David M and Ball S J (2001) Choices of degree or degrees of choice? *Sociology* 35(4): 855–74.

Reid A (1998) *Working Together: Welfare Rights In Primary Care: An Audit of Its Progress.* Wigan and Leigh Specialist Health Promotion Service, Wigan.

Richards H M, Reid M E and Watt G C M (2002) Socioeconomic variations in responses to chest pain: qualitative study. *British Medical Journal* 324: 1308–10.

Roberts J (1996) British nurses at war 1914–1918: ancillary personnel and the battle for registration. *Nursing Research* 45: 167–72.

Roberts K (2001) *Class in Modern Britain.* Palgrave (now Palgrave Macmillan), Basingstoke.

Robertson D (2002) A fair, flexible system is an economic necessity. *The Times Higher Education Supplement* 19 July: 12.

Rogers A and Pilgrim D (1996) *Mental Health Policy in Britain: A Critical Introduction.* Macmillan (now Palgrave Macmillan), London.

Rose D and O'Reilly K (eds) (1997) *Constructing Classes: Towards a New Social Classification for the UK.* ESRC/ONS, Swindon.

Rose D and O'Reilly K (1998) *The ESRC Review of Government Social Classifications: Final Report.* The Stationery Office, London.

Rose G and Marmot M G (1981) Social class and coronary heart disease. *British Medical Journal* 45: 13–19.

Roskell D E (2002) Clinical standards must come before inappropriate blurring of boundaries. *British Medical Journal* eletter 22 January. www.bmj.com/cgi/cletters/324/7330/S23

Royal College of Nursing (RCN) (1994) *Key Activities for Public Health Work In Nursing.* RCN, London.

Royal College of Nursing (RCN) (1996). *Profiling Poverty – A Guide for Nurses in the Community.* RCN, London.

Royal College of Nursing (RCN) (1998) *Working Together for a Healthier Scotland: A Response from the Royal College of Nursing Scottish Board.* RCN, Edinburgh.

Royal College of Nursing (RCN) (2002) *Working Well?* RCN, London.

Royal College of Nursing Defining Nursing Group (2002) *Defining Nursing.* RCN, London.

Royal College of Nursing Presidential Taskforce on Nurse Education (2002) *Quality Education for Quality Care: Position Statement On Nursing Education.* RCN, London.

Royal College of Paediatrics and Child Health (RCPCH) (1999) *Accident and Emergency Services for Children.* RCPCH, London.

Ruskin J (1977 [1851]) *The Nature of Gothic: A Chapter of the Stones of Venice.* Garland, London.

Sadler C (2001) Breath of fresh air. *Nursing Standard* 15(27): 18–19.

Sadler C (2002) Country strife. *Nursing Standard* 16(29): 18–19.

Salmon D and Watson V (2000) *Report of a Scoping Study Analysing Parenting Activities In the South West.* NHSE, Bristol.

Salvage J (1992) The new nursing: empowering patients or empowering nurses? In Robinson J, Gray A and Elkan R (eds) *Policy Issues in Nursing.* Open University Press, Buckingham, pp. 9–23.

Saunders P (1990a) *Social Class and Stratification.* Routledge, London.

Saunders, P (1990b) *A Nation of Home Owners.* London: Unwin Hyman.

Savage M and Egerton M (1997) Social mobility, individual ability and class inequality. *Sociology* 31(4): 645–72.

Scambler G and Higgs P (1999) Stratification, class and health: class relations and health inequalities in high modernity. *Sociology* 33: 275–96.

Scott J (1997) *Corporate Business and Capitalist Classes.* Oxford University Press, Oxford.

Scottish Executive (2001) *Nursing for Health: A Review of the Contribution of Nurses, Midwives and Health Visitors to Improving the Public's Health In Scotland.* The Stationery Office, Edinburgh.

Scottish Office Department of Health (1999) *Towards a Healthier Scotland.* HMSO, Edinburgh.

Scull A (1977) *Decarceration: Community Treatment and the Deviant: A Radical View.* Prentice-Hall, Englewood Cliffs, NJ.

Scull A (1979) *Museums of Madness: The Social Organisation of Insanity in Nineteenth-Century England.* Penguin, London.

Scull A (1996) Asylums: utopias and realities. In Tomlinson D and Carrier J (eds) *Asylum in the Community.* Routledge, London, pp. 7–17.

Sedgwick P (1982) *Psychopolitics.* Pluto Press, London.

Sewell G and Wilkinson B (1992) Someone to watch over me: surveillance, discipline and the just-in-time labour process. *Sociology* 60: 255–66.

Sharp I (ed.) (1999) *Looking to the Future: Making Coronary Heart Disease an Epidemic of the Past.* A Report of the National Heart Forum. The Stationery Office, London.

Shaw M, Dorling D, Gordon D and Davey Smith G (1999) *The Widening Gap: Health Inequalities and Policy In Britain*. The Policy Press, University of Bristol, Bristol.

Shibuya K, Hashimoto H and Yano E (2002) Individual income, income distribution, and self rated health in Japan: cross sectional analysis of a nationally representative sample. *British Medical Journal* 324: 16–19.

Shopland D R, Gerlach K K, Burns D M, Hartman A M and Gibson J T (2001) State specific trends in smoke free workplace policy coverage: the current population survey tobacco use supplement 1993–1999. *Environmental Medicine* 43: 680–6.

Shorter E (1997) *A History of Psychiatry*. John Wiley and Sons, New York.

Siegrist J, Peter R, Junge A, Cremer P and Siedel D (1990) Low status control, high effort at work and ischemic heart disease: prospective evidence from blue-collar men. *Social Science and Medicine* 31: 1127–34.

Silverston H (2001) Latex sensitivity and allergy: raising awareness in Australia. *Australian Journal of Advanced Nursing* 18(3): 40–5.

Skeggs B (1997) *Formations of Class and Gender*. Sage, London.

Sladden S (1979) *Psychiatric Nursing in the Community: A Study of a Working Situation*. Churchill Livingstone, Edinburgh.

Smith D (1976) 1926 remembered and revealed. *Lafur* 2: 26–30.

Smith R (2002) Website Editorial: Doctors and nurses: a new dance? *British Medical Journal* 320: www.bmj.com/cgi/content/full/320/7241/0

Snow J (1936) *On Cholera*. Commonwealth Fund, New York.

Sokejima S and Kagamimori S (1998) Working hours as a risk factor for acute myocardial infarction in Japan: case-control study. *British Medical Journal* 317: 775–80.

Somerville J (1997) Social movement theory, women and the question of interests. *Sociology* 31(4): 673–95.

Stansfeld S, Bosma H, Hemingway H and Marmot M G (1998) Psychosocial work characteristics and social support as predictors of SF36 health functioning: The Whitehall II Study. *Psychosomatic Medicine* 60: 247–55.

Stanworth M (1984) Women and class analysis: a reply to Goldthorpe. *Sociology* 18(2): 159–70.

Statistics (2001) www.dwp.gov.uk/publications/dwp/2001/oppall-third/main/chapter2-17.htm

Steptoe A, Doherty S, Rink E, Kerry S, Kendrick T and Hilton S (1999) Behavioural counselling in general practice for the promotion of healthy behaviour among adults at increased risk of coronary heart disease: randomised trial. *British Medical Journal* 319: 943–8.

Stewart A, Prandy K and Blackburn R M (1980) *Social Stratification and Occupations*. Macmillan (now Palgrave Macmillan), London.

Storey P and Chamberlain R (2001) (Thomas Coram Research Institute, Institute of Education, commissioned by CPAG) *Improving the Take-Up of Free School Meals.* Department for Education and Employment, London.

Sturm R and Gresenz C R (2002) Relations of income inequality and family income to chronic medical conditions and mental health disorders: national survey. *British Medical Journal* 324: 20–3.

Sure Start (2002) www.surestart.gov.uk

Szreter S R S (1984) The genesis of the Registrar General's social classification of occupations. *British Journal of Sociology* 35: 522–46.

Theorell T, Tsutsumi T, Hallqvist J et al. (1998) Decision latitude, job strain and myocardial infarction: a study of working men in Stockholm. *American Journal of Public Health* 88: 382–8.

Thompson D R and Watson R (2001) Editorial: Academic nursing: what is happening to it and where is it going? *Journal of Advanced Nursing* 36(1): 1–2.

Thompson E P (1968) *The Making of the Working Class.* Penguin, Harmondsworth.

Thompson P and Ackroyd S (1995) All quiet on the workplace front? A critique of recent trends in British industrial sociology. *Sociology* 29(4): 615–33.

Thompson P and Bannon E (1985) *Working the System: The Shop Floor and New Technology.* Pluto, London.

Thompson W T, Cupples M E, Sibbett C H, Skan D I and Bradley T (2001) Challenge of culture, conscience and contract to general practitioners' care of their own health: qualitative study. *British Medical Journal* 323: 728–31.

Thomson H, Petticrew M and Morrison D (2001) Health effects of housing improvement: systematic review of intervention studies. *British Medical Journal* 323: 187–90.

Tod A M, Read C, Lacey A and Abbott J (2001) Barriers to uptake of services for coronary heart disease: qualitative study. *British Medical Journal* 323: 214–17.

Touraine A (1995) Sociology and the study of society. In Joyce P (ed.) *Class.* Oxford University Press, Oxford, pp. 83–7.

Townsend P, Davidson N and Whitehead M (eds) (1988a) *Inequalities in Health: The Black Report and The Health Divide.* Penguin, Harmondsworth.

Townsend P, Phillimore P and Beattie A (1988b) *Health and Deprivation: Inequality and the North.* London, Croom Helm.

Tumin M (1964) Some principles of stratification: a critical analysis. In Coser L A and Rosenberg B (eds) *Sociological Theory.* Collier-Macmillan, London.

Uehata T (1991) Long working hours and occupational stress-related cardiovascular attacks among middle-aged workers in Japan. *Journal of Human Ergonomics* 20: 147–53.

United Kingdom Central Council for Nursing, Midwifery and Health Visiting (UKCC) (1986) *Project 2000: A New Preparation for Practice.* UKCC, London.

United Kingdom Central Council for Nursing, Midwifery and Health Visiting (UKCC) (1999) *Fitness for Practice: The UKCC Commission for Nursing and Midwifery Education*. Chair, Sir Leonard Peach (The Peach Report). UKCC, London.

Universities UK (2002) *Social Class and Participation*. Report commissioned by Universities UK and prepared by the European Access Network at the University of Westminster. Universities UK, London.

Vahter M, Berglund M, Akesson A and Liden C (2002) Metals and women's health. *Environmental Research* 88(3): 145–55.

Veitch D (1995) *Prescribing Citizen's Advice: An Evaluation of the Work of the Citizens' Advice Bureaux with Health and Social Services in Birmingham*. Birmingham District Citizens' Advice Bureaux Ltd, Birmingham.

Virtanen P, Vahtera J, Kivimäki M, Pentti J and Ferrie J (2002) Employment security and health. *Journal of Epidemiology Community Health* 56: 569–74.

Wadsworth M E J (1986) Serious illness in childhood and its association with later-life achievement. In Wilkinson R G (ed.) *Class and Health: Research and Longitudinal Data*. Tavistock, London.

Wadsworth M E J (1991) *The Imprint of Time: Childhood, History and Adult Life*. Clarendon Press, Oxford.

Wadsworth M E J (1996) Family and education as determinants of health. In Blane D, Brunner E and Wilkinson R (eds) *Health and Social Organisation*. Routledge, London, pp. 152–70.

Wadsworth M E J and Kuh D J L (1997) Childhood influences on adult health: a review of recent work from the British 1946 national birth cohort study, the MRC National Survey of Health and Development. *Pediatric and Perinatal Epidemiology* 11: 2–20.

Wamala S P, Mittleman M A, Schenck-Gustafsson and Orth-Gomer K (1999) Potential explanations for the educational gradient in coronary heart disease: a population-based case–control study of Swedish women. *American Journal of Public Health* 89(3): 315–21.

Warner R (1985) *Recovery From Schizophrenia: Psychiatry and Political Economy*. Second edition. Routledge, London.

Warr P and Jackson P R (1987) Adapting to the unemployed role: a longitudinal investigation. *Social Science and Medicine* 25: 1219–24.

Wasling C (1999) Role of the cardioprotective diet in preventing coronary heart disease. *British Journal of Nursing* 8(18): 1242–8.

Waters A (2002) Countdown to the final evaluation. *Nursing Standard* 16(50): 12–13.

Waters M (1997) Inequality after class. In Owen D (ed.) *Sociology After Postmodernism*. Sage, London.

Watterson A (1999) Why we still have 'old' epidemics and 'endemics' in occupational health: policy and practice failures and some possible solutions. In Daykin N and Doyal L (eds) *Health and Work: Critical Perspectives.* Macmillan (now Palgrave Macmillan), London, pp. 107–26.

Webb C (2002) The international contribution of feminist thinking to the development of nursing. Plenary lecture, 8 April, RCN Annual International Research Society Conference, Exeter.

Webb J (1999) Work and the new public service class? *Sociology* 33(4): 747–66.

Weber M (1945) (Gerth H and Mills C W (eds)) *From Max Weber.* Routledge, London.

Weber M (1968) (Roth R and Wittich C (eds)) *Economy and Society.* Bedminster Press, New York.

Weber M (1995 [1978]) Max Weber on class. In Joyce P (ed.) *Class.* Oxford University Press, Oxford, pp. 31–40.

Webster C (1996) *Government and Health Care: Volume II. The National Health Service 1958–1979.* HMSO, London.

Westergaard J H (1995) *Who Gets What?* Polity Press, Cambridge.

Whitaker S, Wynn P and Williams N (2002) Occupational health teaching for pre-registration nursing students. *Nurse Education Today* 22(2): 152–8.

White S (1991) *Political Theory and Postmodernism.* Cambridge University Press, Cambridge.

Whitehouse C R (1985) Effect of distance from surgery on consultation rates in an urban practice. *British Medical Journal* 290: 359–62.

Whiteman M C, Deary I J, Lee A J and Fowkes F G R (1997) Submissiveness and protection from coronary heart disease in the general population: Edinburgh Artery Study. *Lancet* 23 August: 541–5.

Whiting M (1998) Focus on community children's nursing. *British Journal of Community Nursing* 3(4): 186–90.

Whiting M (2000) 1888–1988: 100 years of community children's nursing. In Muir J and Sidey A (eds) *Textbook of Community Children's Nursing.* Baillière Tindall/RCN, London.

Wiles R (1997) Empowering practice nurses in the follow-up of patients with established heart disease: lessons from patients' experience. *Journal of Advanced Nursing* 26(4): 729–35.

Wilkinson R G (1992) Income distribution and life expectancy. *British Medical Journal* 304: 165–8.

Wilkinson R G (1994) Health, redistribution and growth. In Glyn A and Milliband D (eds) *Paying for Inequality: The Economic Cost of Social Injustice.* Rivers Oram Press, London.

Wilkinson R G (1996a) *Unhealthy Societies: The Afflictions of Inequality.* Routledge, London.

Wilkinson R G (1996b) How can secular improvements in life expectancy be explained? In Blane D, Brunner E and Wilkinson R G (eds) *Health and Social Organisation: Towards a Health Policy for the 21st Century.* Routledge, London, pp. 109–22.

Wilkinson R G (1999) Putting the picture together: Prosperity, redistribution, health and welfare. In Marmot M and Wilkinson R G (eds) *Social Determinants of Health.* Oxford University Press, Oxford, pp. 256–74.

Wilkinson R G (2002) Income inequality and population health: letter. *British Medical Journal* 324: 978.

Wilkinson R G and Marmot M (1998) (eds) *Social Determinants of Health: The Solid Facts.* WHO Regional Office for Europe, Copenhagen.

Wilkinson R G and Miers M (1999) Power and professions. In Wilkinson G and Miers M (eds) *Power and Nursing Practice.* Macmillan (now Palgrave Macmillan), Basingstoke, pp. 24–36.

Wilkinson R G, Kawachi I and Kennedy B (1998) Mortality, the social environment, crime and violence. *Sociology of Health and Illness* 20: 578–97.

Williams S, Michie S and Pattani S (1998) *Improving the Health of the NHS Workforce: Report of the Partnership On the Health of the NHS Workforce.* Nuffield Trust, London.

Willis P (1977) *Learning to Labour: How Working Class Kids Get Working Class Jobs.* Columbia University Press, New York.

Winter J M (1985) *The Great War and the British People.* Macmillan (now Palgrave Macmillan), London.

Winter J M (1988) Public health and the extension of life expectancy 1901–60. In Keynes M (ed.) *The Political Economy of Health and Welfare.* Cambridge University Press, Cambridge, pp. 109–32.

Witz A (1992) *Professions and Patriarchy.* Routledge, London.

Wolf Z R (1996) Bowel management and nursing's hidden work. *Nursing Times* 92(21): 26–8.

Wolfensberger W (1972) *Normalization.* National Institute of Mental Retardation, Toronto.

Wolfson M, Kaplan G, Lynch J, Ross N, Backlund E, Gravelle H and Wilkinson R G (1999) Relation between income inequality and mortality: empirical demonstration. Diminishing returns to aggregate level studies. Two pathways, but how much do they diverge? *British Medical Journal* 319: 953–7.

World Bank (1993) *The East Asian Miracle.* Oxford University Press, Oxford.

World Health Organisation (WHO) (1985) *Targets for Health for All: Targets in Support of the European Regional Strategy for Health for All by the Year 2000.* WHO Regional Office for Europe, Copenhagen.

Worsnip J (1990) A re-evaluation of the problem of surplus women in nineteenth century England. *Women's Studies International Forum* 13: 21–31.

Wright C (1996) Top of the class. *Nursing Times* 92(50): 16–17.

Wright E O (1979) *Class Structure and Income Determination.* Academic Press, New York.

Wright E O (1985) *Classes*. Verso, London.

Wright E O (1997) *Class Counts*. Cambridge University Press, Cambridge.

Wright L, Jolly K, Speller V and Smith H (1999) The success of an integrated care programme for patients with ischaemic heart disease: the practice nurses' perspective of SHIP. *Journal of Clinical Nursing* 8(5): 519–26.

Wright R L, Wiles R A and Moher M (2001) Patients' and practice nurses' perceptions of secondary preventive care for established ischaemic heart disease: a qualitative study. *Journal of Clinical Nursing* 10(2): 180–8.

Name index

Subject index